W0106389

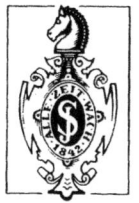

S. Fregert   H.-J. Bandmann

Patch Testing

Published on behalf of the
International Contact Dermatitis Research Group

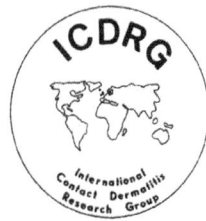

H.-J. Bandmann, Munich, West Germany
C. D. Calnan, London, United Kingdom
E. Cronin, London, United Kingdom
S. Fregert, Lund, Sweden
N. Hjorth, Copenhagen, Denmark
B. Magnusson, Malmö, Sweden
H. I. Maibach, San Francisco, Calif., USA
K. E. Malten, Nijmegen, Netherlands
C. L. Meneghini, Bari, Italy
V. Pirilä, Helsinki, Finland
D. S. Wilkinson, High Wycombe, United Kingdom

With 3 Figures and 17 Tables

Springer-Verlag

Berlin Heidelberg New York 1975

Professor Dr. S. Fregert
University of Lund
Section of Occupational Dermatology
University Hospital
Lund/Sweden

Professor D. H.-J. Bandmann
Dermatologische Klinik der Universität
8000 München 740
Kölner Platz 1

Original title of the German edition:
Bandmann/Fregert: Epicutantestung. (Kliniktaschenbücher)

ISBN-13:978-3-540-07229-4   e-ISBN-13:978-3-642-66110-5
DOI: 10.1007/978-3-642-66110-5

Library of Congress Cataloging in Publication Data. Bandmann, Hans-Jürgen.
Patch testing. Translation of Epicutantestung. In German ed. Bandmann's
name appears first on title page. Bibliography: p.   . Includes index. 1. Skin.
I. Fregert, Sigfrid, joint author. II. International Contact Dermatitis Research
Group. III. Title. [DNLM: 1. Skin diseases—Diagnosis. 2. Skin tests. WR140
F858e]. RC587.S6B3213 616.9'7'075 75-2387

Contents

1. General Aspects

1.1 Introduction

The patch test (epicutaneous test) and photo patch test are used to clarify the etiology and diagnosis of allergic as well as light-potentiated contact dermatitis. The patch test must be correlated with historic data and physical examination.

Contact dermatitis constitutes a significant proportion (5%–15%) of the diseases at dermatologic clinics.

If the results are to be reliable, patch tests should be performed properly and the technique should not be varied in an arbitrary manner. The examiner should adhere strictly to the standard procedure so as to understand its possibilities and its limitations.

Interpretation of the actual patch test reactions places high demands on the experience and skill of the examiner and on his knowledge of chemistry and pharmacology.

This monograph is concerned only with the patch test method used to demonstrate the existence of contact allergy and light-potentiated contact allergy. It does not describe the "prophetic patch test" ("predictive patch test"), which is used to demonstrate the sensitizing capacity of a substance.

The *terminology* in the text is that recommended by the International Contact Dermatitis Research Group. (In this book dermatitis = eczema.)

1.2 Historic Development

Joseph Jadassohn devised the epicutaneous test. In 1895 he tested a syphilitic patient who developed a cutaneous eruption after treatment with mercury ointment.

He applied mercury to the patient's upper arm, covered it with adhesive tape, and found that the subsequent reaction extended from the wrist to the shoulder and over half of the chest. The patient was regarded as reacting abnormally to mercury, having what was known at that time as an idiosyncrasy. The term *allergy* was coined by von Pirquet in 1906. Such reactions had previously been seen after local applications containing quinine, iodoform, or

1

mercury, but none of the patients affected had been tested to see if they responded abnormally to these substances.

The term *patch test* was proposed by Cooke (1916).

Bloch, in Zurich, elaborated the method and introduced the use of a standard series of seven test substances (turpentine, formaldehyde, tincture of arnica, sublimate, quinine, iodoform, and *Primula obconica*). The method is often called Jadassohn-Bloch's patch test.

1.3 Principles of Patch Testing

The purpose of the patch test is to detect contact allergy.

It is performed by applying the suspected substance in a standardized fashion and in the correct concentration to normal skin. If an eczematous response is elicited, the person probably has a contact allergy to the tested substance.

In contact allergy, the entire skin reacts, but only certain areas of the body provide background information, making them suitable for patch testing. Several test substances may be applied simultaneously. Patch testing is an artificial procedure and is not a true reproduction of the contact that occurs in a person's normal environment, where exposure often includes a number of factors that influence percutaneous absorption of the substance in question. To facilitate absorption of the test substances, they are generally applied under occlusion.

Contact allergy varies in intensity from one person to another. To produce a positive reaction, the threshold value of sensitivity must be exceeded. Absorption varies with the technique used and with other conditions, such as temperature, moisture, and season, at the time of testing.

Patch testing is therefore a relatively crude bioassay method for determining contact allergy, which is not an all-or-none reaction, but occurs in all degrees of intensity. The test reaction may therefore be negative in a patient in whom a high concentration, or long-term exposure, or both, in a habitual environment might produce allergic contact dermatitis. On the other hand, the test reaction may be positive, but the clinical contact may be short and the allergen may be present in a concentration too low to produce contact dermatitis.

The appearance of the patch-test reaction may differ considerably from that of the contact dermatitis elicited by the same allergen; possible reasons for such differences include a change in the clinical picture of the dermatitis after its onset and the action of additional chemical or physical factors on the skin.

1.4 Indications

The range of indications for patch testing varies widely among dermatologists. Some feel that patch testing does not provide information over and above that obtained from the history and examination of the patient, whereas others use patch testing not only in patients with suspected allergic contact dermatitis, but in almost every patient with dermatitis.

The range of indications used by each dermatologist depends on his opinion of the value of the information obtained balanced against the risk of patch-test sensitization.

The number of allergic positive reactions and the percentage of such reactions that can be explained by history and physical examination vary with the range of indications. They also depend on whether or not a standard series is used, the choice of substances for such series, the thoroughness with which the patient's history is taken, and the consequent use of supplementary test substances.

The following guidelines for patch-test indications are recommended.

Patch testing is indicated in suspected allergic contact dermatitis when the cause is unknown or uncertain. When the history and examination focus on a particularly well-known allergen, the indication for testing may be weaker. This would apply to the typical brief eruptions that occur after known contact with plants, such as *Primula obconica* or poison ivy. If the clinical course is prolonged, patch testing may be indicated even if one or several sensitizers are known to be the major cause of the dermatitis, because a coexisting but less obvious allergy may be delaying healing.

However, it must be emphasized that *clinical impressions can be misleading.* In many cases of allergic contact dermatitis contact allergy is not suspected. The history may not contain any reference to an allergen, especially if the offending allergen is a ubiquitous one encountered by everybody, such as chromate, nickel, rubber, dyes, or perfumes. The *clinical picture* is not always so obvious as in nickel dermatitis under a brassiere clasp. The lesions may be modified by the superimposed action of irritants or concomitant allergens, as in most cases of *hand eczema*, as well as by therapy and by spontaneous improvement.

Allergic contact dermatitis may simulate other varieties of dermatitis and eruptions, such as *atopic dermatitis*, and *nummular eczema* may in fact be cement dermatitis. *Primula obconica* can cause a clinical picture simulating *seborrheic dermatitis.*

Experience shows that *stasis dermatitis* is often complicated by contact sensitivity to topical pharmaceutical preparations, although clinical features may vary. Allergic contact dermatitis due to certain film developers that contain azo compounds may cause a *lichenoid dermatitis*, and rubber, particularly from tires and tubes, can simulate *Trichophyton rubrum infection* of the palms.

The indication for patch testing becomes wider if contact with a suspected allergen is unavoidable, especially if a change of occupation or insurance compensation depends upon it. The same applies when it might be difficult or troublesome to avoid an allergen, such as wearing chromium-free shoes or nonallergenic stockings.

The risk of *patch-test sensitization* with some substances, e.g., chlorpromazine, should be considered and balanced against the need for a patch test.

If patch testing is indicated, the investigation should *include both a standard series* (routine series, battery) and *additional substances* suggested by the history. A standard series can, however, sometimes be omitted in cases of typical contact dermatitis due to plants, topical drugs, cosmetics, or industrial chemicals. If patch testing with the suspected allergens gives negative reactions and the dermatitis is prolonged, routine patch testing should be performed.

Indications for photo patch testing: see chap. 5.4.

1.5 Contraindications

Existing *acute or widespread dermatitis* is a relative contraindication because the dermatitis may flare up or elicit nonspecific test reactions or both.

The intended *test site should have been clear of dermatitis for at least 2 weeks* and preferably a month.

Corrosives in high concentration and substances with *systemic toxic* effects, especially pesticides or new substances from research laboratories, the hazards of which are unknown, should not be used for patch testing in routine clinics.

Systemic treatment with less than 20 mg prednisolone per day, as a rule, does not significantly inhibit an allergic test reaction in a hypersensitive person. Antihistamines do not inhibit patch-test reactions.

2. Test Technique

2.1 Principles of the Technique

Selected substances are diluted to the correct concentration by incorporating them in a suitable vehicle. This preparation is applied to the test unit, which is made up of a filter-paper disk covered by an impermeable sheet. The test unit *is applied to the skin* and fixed in position with *occlusive adhesive tape*, which is left *in situ for 2 days*; it is then removed and the first *reading* is *recorded*.

The following details are recommended:

2.2 Test Substances

Substances for a standard series should ideally be chemically identified and as pure as possible. Most patch testing is done with standard materials available commercially. Other substances such as turpentine, i.e., the composition of which varies and is not fully known, should be purchased in large quantities so

Table 1. Characteristics of test substances (examples)

Chemically defined substances	Natural mixtures	Artificial mixtures
Halogen hydroxyquinolines	Lanolin	Paraben mix
Benzocaine	Balsam of Peru	Thiram mix
Formaldehyde	Tincture of benzoin	PPD mix
Potassium dichromate	Colophony	Naphthyl mix
Cobalt chloride	Turpentine	Carba mix
Mafenide (sulfamylon)	Coal tar	Commercial cosmetic and pharmaceutical preparations
Neomycin	Wood tar	
Nickel sulfate		
Parabens		
p-Phenylenediamine		
Primin		

Table 2. Mixtures of test substances

Symbols:
□ 5 ml in aluminium tubes
■ 10 ml in aluminium tubes
▲ 5 ml in plastic syringes
▼ 2·5 ml in plastic syringes

Firm	No.	Trade name	%	Vehicle	Symbol
I. *Paraben mixture*					
1. Hermal	21	Parabens	1	Petrolatum	□
2. Hollister-Stier		Paraben mix (P)	15	Petrolatum	▼
		Ethyl paraben	5		
		Methyl paraben	5		
		Propyl paraben	5		
3. Dr. Sasse	10	*p*-Hydroxybenzoates	10	Petrolatum	■
		Methylparaben	5		
		Propylparaben	5		
4. Trolab	0012	Parabens	15	Petrolatum	▲
		Ethylparaben	3		
		Benzylparaben	3		
		Butylparaben	3		
		Methylparaben	3		
		Propylparaben	3		
II. *Rubber mixture*					
1. Hollister-Stier		Rubber mix (R)	2	Petrolatum	▼
		Mercaptobenzthiazol	1		
		Tetramethylthiuram-disulfide	1		
2. Trolab	0022	Mercapto mix;	1	Petrolatum	▲
		Mercaptobenzthiazol	0·25		
		N-Cyclohexyl-benzthiazylsulf-enamide	0·25		
		Dibenzthiazyl disulfide	0·25		
		Morpholinylmercapto-benzthiazole	0·25		
	0023	Thiram mix:	1	Petrolatum	▲
		Tetraethyl-thiuram disulfide	0·25		
		Tetramethyl-thiurammono sulfide	0·25		
		Tetraethy-thiuram disulfide	0·25		
		Dipentamethylen-thiuram disulfide	0·25		
	0024	PPD mix	0·60	Petrolatum	▲
		Phenylcyclohexyl-*p*-phenylenediamine	0·25		
		Isopropylamino-diphenylamine	0·10		

Table 2—continued

Firm	No.	Trade name	%	Vehicle	Symbol
		Diphenyl-*p*-phenyl-			
		enediamine	0·25		
	0025	Naphthyl-mix	1	Petrolatum	▲
		Phenyl-*β*-			
		naphthylamine	0·5		
		Di-*β*-naphthyl-*p*-			
		phenylenediamine	0·5		
	1020	Carba mix	3	Petrolatum	▲
		1,3-Diphenyl-			
		guanidine	1		
		Zinc diethyldithio-			
		carbamate	1		
		Zinc dibutyldithio-			
		carbamate	1		
III. *Caine mixture*					
1. Hollister-Stier		Caine mix C	9	Petrolatum	▼
		Ethoform			
		(Benzocaine)	5		
		Cinchocaine			
		(Nupercaine)	1		
		Triprilenamine			
		(Pyribensamine)	2		
		Cyclomethycaine			
		(Surfacaine)	1		
2. Trolab	0404	Caine mix	8	Petrolatum	▲
		Cinchocaine–HCl	1		
		Tetracaine–HCl	1		
		Cyclomethycaine			
		(Surfacaine)	1		
		Ethoform			
		(Benzocaine)	5		
IV. *Pharmaceutical mixture*					
1. Hollister-Stier		Medimix (M)	4·2	Petrolatum	▼
		Nitrofural (Furacin)	0·2		
		Methapyrilen HCl			
		(Histadyl)	1		
		Iodochlorohydroxy-			
		quinoline (vioform)	3		
V. *Wood tar mixture*					
1. Hermal	9	Wood tar	10	Petrolatum	□
2. Trolab	001	Wood tars	1	Petrolatum	▲
		Pine	3		
		Beech	3		
		Juniper	3		
		Birch	3		

that laboratory requirements can be covered for several years, thus avoiding changes in composition.

Well-defined substances, such as metals and drugs, should be of *analytical quality* (Table 1). Rubber chemicals, on the other hand, should be of *technical quality*, because the actual allergen in *p*-phenylenediamine rubber derivatives is not known.

Besides the substances in the standard series, the test laboratory should have a selection of other identified substances, which can be used for additional tests (Tables 17a,b,c, see page 457).

Technical products, cosmetics, and drugs should be available, but it is wiser to use the patient's own preparations and thus avoid any differences in composition due to changes in the manufacturers' formulation or alterations during storage.

When the sensitizers are known, as in the case of the more common drugs, cosmetics, and possibly, also industrial chemicals, they should be available for testing.

Most test substances, both analytical and technical, are commercially available.

Some substances can also be purchased in the correct concentrations and vehicles as ready-made test preparations (Table 17a).

Certain substances may be used in *mixtures* (Table 2), provided they do not interact with one another.

Some products brought by patients must *first be prepared* in various ways:

Solid materials, such as plastic, leather, wood, or bark, may give false-positive reactions owing to irregular and excessive pressure of the solid piece of test material. This can be avoided by pulverizing it with a saw or an electric drill, scissors, or a file; a curette can be used to obtain specimens from different parts of boots and shoes. Soft material, such as rubber, may be applied in thin, even sheets. Textiles can be applied as they are. Solid materials should be moistened with water.

Plants brought by the patient should each be wrapped separately in aluminium foil or envelopes to prevent them from contaminating one another during transport. Testing with *Primula obconica* can be standardized in selected cases by using an extract or, preferably, pure primin applied to filter paper patches and stored in aluminium foil (Table 17a). Leaves, flowers, and stalks can be cut into thin slices.

Acid and alkaline products may sometimes be made suitable by neutralizing them with sodium hydroxide $(0 \cdot 1 – 0 \cdot 01 \, N)$ or soda, or hydrochloric acid $(1 – 0 \cdot 1 \, M)$, or acetic acid, respectively. Alternatively, they may be dissolved in a buffer solution.

Certain products, such as nail polish and hair lotions, may be applied if *all of the irritant solvent is first removed* by evaporation, either at room temperature or at a higher temperature $(50° – 80°C)$, in a sand bath or in a vacuum.

8

Extraction with acetone or absolute alcohol at higher temperatures (50°–80°C) in a sand bath for 15–30 minutes may be useful when materials such as textiles, rubber, shoe lining or sole, plants, and others, are being tested.

2.3 Vehicles

Most substances, mixtures, and products are unsuitable for direct application to the skin because of their irritant effect. They should be diluted to a suitable concentration in a proper vehicle. Many substances can be dissolved in *water*, e.g., metal salts, formaldehyde. Other substances must be dissolved in *absolute ethyl alcohol, acetone, isobutylketone, methylethylketone (MEK), butyl- or ethylacetate, olive oil, or liquid paraffin.*

Solvents such as chloroform, white spirit, benzene, toluene, oil of turpentine, carbon disulfide, and petrol (benzene, gasoline) are irritants and should not be used as vehicles. Sometimes it is necessary to use an irritant solvent to dissolve glues and plastics. The solution obtained can then be diluted to a nonirritant concentration with, e.g., olive oil.

Lanolin (or Eucerin and wool alcohols) should not be used as vehicles, since many patients are sensitized to these compounds.

When test substances are dissolved in an organic solvent there is the possibility that their concentrations will increase during storage due to evaporation of the solvent. In addition, certain substances tend to change due to oxidation, and ethyl alcohol is readily reduced at pH < 7.

Therefore, in recent years *yellow petrolatum* Vaseline has been widely used to avoid these effects and to facilitate occlusion. It is thought to give more reliable results. Bleached white petrolatum should not be used because occasionally it may be irritating.

The test substance should first be ground in a porcelain or agate mortar and should then be put into a well, prepared in a weighed amount of petrolatum in a glass vessel. A few drops of a suitable solvent are then added. To ensure even distribution, the mixture must then be stirred for 5 minutes with a glass rod.

Weighing petrolatum is troublesome, but it can be facilitated by first melting it and then pouring it into polypropylene or polyethylene syringes. A weight of 10 g corresponds to about 12 ml (check petrolatum in question). A suitable batch of petrolatum can be stored and squirted into the mixing vessel as required. Petrolatum should not be melted after the test substance has been added. Filling syringes or aluminium tubes with the test preparations can be facilitated by using a glass rod.

2.4 Storage

Organic substances should be stored in sealed packages, some under refrigeration and some in a well-ventilated cupboard. Hygroscopic substances should

9

be stored in packages with a water-absorbing substance (usually silica gel), in the same way as certain drugs.

Substances that may change when exposed to light should be kept *in amber-colored glassware.*

Material brought by patients preferably should be stored in polyethylene bags labeled with their name and code number. Some test solutions containing water or organic solvents should be renewed every 2–4 weeks because of the risk of degradation and change in concentration. Solutions are kept in pipette glass bottles. Rubber pipette caps should not be used because the solution may become contaminated with rubber chemicals.

Petrolatum preparations should be kept in 10-ml *propylene or polyethylene syringes,* which should not have rubber plungers. Most of these preparations can be stored for one year.

The test preparations should *preferably be kept in the dark.*

2.5 Concentrations

The concentration of the test substance is of fundamental importance in the results of the test. Unduly high concentrations can cause false-positive reactions and may even cause test sensitization. On the other hand, if the concentration is too low, the test may give a false-negative reaction. Furthermore, the proper concentration depends not only on the substance, but also on the vehicle and the patch-test unit. Thus, the concentration used must be lower if occlusion is complete.

Irritant reactions to substances in the standard series described here are rare, but substances used sporadically are likely to cause such reactions. However, even standard test substances that do not normally produce irritant reactions in the concentrations used routinely may *produce false-positive reactions in some substances and false-negative responses in others under certain circumstances.* The choice of concentration with a given test technique is therefore a question of compromise. Systematic studies to find the most suitable concentration with different vehicles and test materials have not been performed on a sufficiently large number of materials. The concentration must, therefore, be selected on the basis of clinical experience, which may, however, also be misleading.

The choice of concentration of unknown substances and products, especially industrial ones, is difficult. Because of wide individual variations in skin irritability, it would be desirable to patch test a minimum of 20 healthy volunteers. However, for practical reasons this is often impossible and, furthermore, there is always the risk of patch-test sensitization to unknown substances.

It might be advisable to perform an open test with different concentrations first. The suitable concentration for many substances is 0.1%–2% in closed

Table 3. Standard test series (Europe) recommended by ICDRG

I			II			III		
No.	Test subst.	%	No.	Test subst.	%	No.	Test subst.	%
1	Neomycin		7	Epoxy resin	1	13	p-Phenylene	
	sulfate	20	8	Chinoform	5		diamine (PPD)	2
2	Potassium		9	Cobalt		14	Naphthyl mix	1
	dichromate	0·5		chloride	1	15	Colophony	20
3	Wool alcohols	30	10	Balsam of Peru	25	16	PPD mix	0·6
4	Mercapto mix	1	11	Thiram mix	1	17	Turpentine	
5	Benzocaine	5	12	Parabens			peroxides	0·3
6	Nickel sulfate	5		(mix)	15	18	Formaldehyde	2·5

Vehicles: No. 1–16 petrolatum: No. 17 olive oil: No. 18 water.
Mix: see Table 4 (Trolab).

patch testing. Most drugs and cosmetics can be used as they are, but there is a risk of false-negative reactions.

2.6 Selection of Test Substances

Although thousands of substances have been described as contact allergens, most cases of allergic contact dermatitis are probably caused by 20–30 sub-

Table 3a. Standard test series recommended by North American Contact Dermatitis Group

I		II	
No.	%	No.	%
1 Neomycin sulfate	20	6 Thiomersal	0·1
2 Ammoniated mercury	1	7 Mercapto mix	1
3 Potassium dichromate	0·5	8 Balsam of Peru	25
4 Ethylenediamine	1	9 Turpentine peroxides	0·3
5 Nickel sulfate	2·5	10 p-Phenylenediamine	1

III		IV	
No.	%	No.	%
11 Thiram mix	1	16 Parabens	15
12 Wool alcohols	30	17 Epoxy resins	1
13 Carba mix	3	18 PPD mix	0·6
14 Caine mix	8	19 p-tert. butylphenol	12
15 Formaldehyde	2	20 Naphthyl mix	1
		21 PCMX	1

Vehicles: petrolatum, No. 9 olive oil, No. 15 water.
PCMX Chloroxylenol, widely used antiseptic preservative in the United States.

stances. In some patients with allergic contact dermatitis, the offending allergen can be suspected, but other substances occur in practically all environments so that nearly everyone is exposed to them. It is therefore difficult to detect the actual allergen from the patient's history. Relatively few cases of allergic contact dermatitis are so typical they can be recognized from the clinical features.

Table 4. Test series for dermatitis of the lower leg

No.		%
1	Neomycin sulfate	20
2	Chinoform	5
3	Benzocaine	5
4	Wool alcohols	30
5	Balsam of Peru	25
6	Chlorquinaldol	5
7	Parabens (mix)	15
8	Eucerin anhydrous	100
9	Colophony	20

Vehicle: petrolatum.

For these reasons the use of a *standard test series* (battery) has become common. Many of the standard substances are common to all industrialized countries (Table 3, 3a), but *the selection must always be adapted to the local occurrence* of particular industrial products, drugs, and plants.

Testing with only a standard battery is not sufficient. Investigation should be extended to include substances suggested by the patient's history, and, occasionally, it may be useful to try an additional battery, such as topical-drugs or substances known to cause dermatitis of the leg (Table 4).

2.7 Test Material

The *patch-test unit* to which the test substance is applied should consist of a filter paper disk, so that it can absorb solutions, although this is not necessary for petrolatum preparations. All filter papers should be of uniform size, e.g., 1 cm in diameter, to achieve good occlusion. To prevent substances from permeating the adhesive tape, the patch-test disk should be covered with a larger piece of material, which is impermeable to water and organic solvents. Hence, cellophane and cellulose acetate should not be used.

This covering material should be inert and should not contain any chemical capable of producing skin reactions. A suitable material is aluminium foil lined with polyethylene that does not contain an antioxidant. In addition, the material should preferably be nontransparent so that it will be suitable for photo patch testing.

The filter paper disk should be attached, but not glued, to the impermeable covering sheet.

The *impermeable sheet* should overlap the filter paper disk by at least 0.5 cm so that the area surrounding the actual test site will be protected from possible reaction to the adhesive tape.

The test material should be easy to handle and the patches should be placed at equal and adequate distances from one another (Fig. 1).

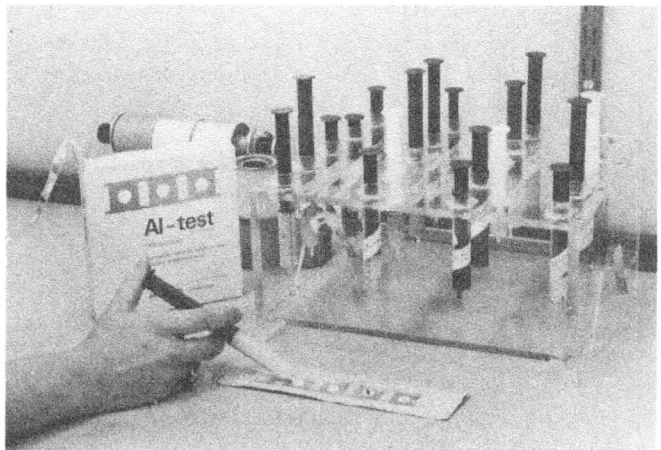

Fig. 1. Application of test preparation (with petrolatum as vehicle, in plastic syringe) to the test patch. (Al test, IMECO Astra Agency, Sweden.)

Before the test substances are applied to the filter paper disks, the patch-test unit should be placed on strips of adhesive tape cut to suitable lengths.

2.8 Application of Test Substances to Patch

The filter-paper patch should be saturated with the test solution, care being taken that no surplus contaminates the surrounding impermeable sheet.

Most solvents begin to evaporate even before the patch is applied to the skin. The concentration of the substance may therefore rise to 100%, so that the amount applied is important. The patch is presumably moistened by the skin during the test period.

13

Table 5. "Para substances"

I. *p*-aminobenzoic acid derivatives

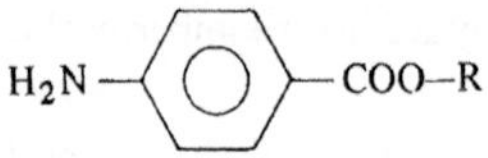

H_2N—⬡—COO—R

R = —CH_2—CH_3

Benzocaine (Ethoform): anesthetic agent
ethyl-4-aminobenzoate

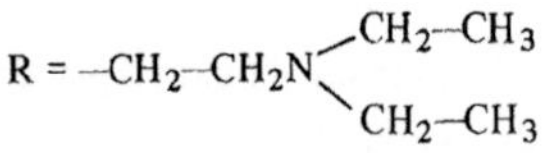

R = —CH_2—CH_2N⟨ CH_2—CH_3 / CH_2—CH_3

Procaine: Local anesthetic agent
2-diethylamino-ethyl ester of
    4-aminobenzoic acid

R = —CH_2—CH—N⟨ CH_2—CH_3 / CH_2—CH_3
               |
             CH_2
               |
             CH_2—CH_3
               |
             CH_3

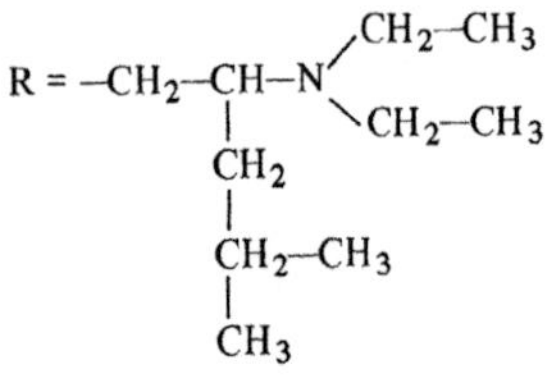

Leucinocaine: Local anesthetic agent

2-diethylamino-4-methyl-
    -pentylester of 4-aminobenzoic acid

R = —H

p-aminobenzoic acid: sunscreen

II. Aniline derivatives

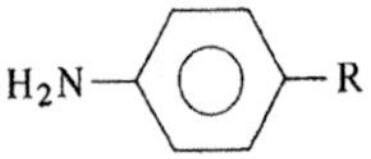

H_2N—⬡—R

R = —NH_2

p-phenylenediamine   Dye

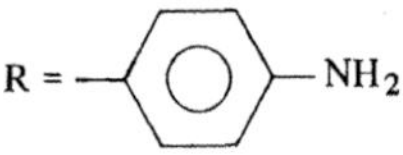

R = —⬡—NH_2

benzidine   Dye

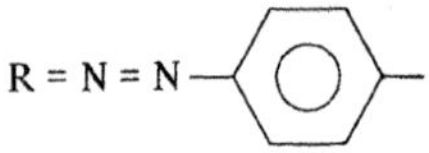

R = N = N—⬡—

p-aminoazobenzene   Dye

R = —N—⬡—

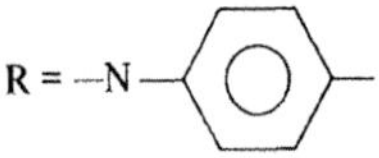

p-aminodiphenylamine   Dye

III. Para substances

Sulfamylon   Antimicrobial preparation
Sulfatolamide   Antimicrobial preparation
Tetracaine   Local anesthetic agent
N-phenyl-cyclohexyl-*p*-phenylenediamine   Rubber chemical
Diphenyl-*p*-phenylenediamine   Rubber chemical
Isoporopylaminodiphenylamine   Rubber chemical
p-Toluylenediamine   Dye
Isobutyl-*p*-aminobenzoate   Sunscreen

When the substances are applied *in petrolatum, the concentration remains constant* and the amount used is therefore of less importance. For practical reasons, a syringe should be used to apply a strip of about one-half the diameter of the patch. The strip should be 1·5–2 mm thick, which can be obtained with a Record syringe; the Luer syringe gives a somewhat thicker strip but can be fitted with an adapter.

Substances that cross-react or often produce simultaneous reactions should not be placed close to one another (Table 5).

A "Patch Test Antigen Dispenser" has been devised, which consists of a metal frame into which up to five metal trays, each holding five glass or polypropylene syringes can be slotted. The distance between individual syringes is 3·6 cm.

2.9 Adhesive Tape

The adhesive tape should be impermeable, so as to secure good occlusion, and about 5 cm wide; it should have *good adhesive properties*.

Reactions to the adhesive tape are relatively common and are of both the allergic and irritant type. Occlusive tapes that adhere well tend to cause reactions more often than do porous tapes.

Patients who report intolerance to adhesive tape should preferably be pretested for 2 days with various types of adhesive tape applied directly to an area not smaller than 5 × 5 cm.

Irritant reactions to tape are liable to occur in patients with widespread or acute dermatitis e.g., stasis eczema of the lower leg. Irritant reactions are not uncommon in the aged and in patients with a dry skin. Some patients develop *folliculitis* and others a *sweat-retention* reaction under the tape.

Allergic reactions are caused mainly by colophony (rosin) and by antioxidants. Modern tapes based on acrylic resins are generally less irritating, but their plasticizers and antioxidants may cause allergic reactions. Allergic reactions to some brands of acrylic tapes have not been reported.

2.10 Application on the Skin

The test units should be placed on the *back* in vertical rows over the scapulae and not over the vertebral column. The upper end of the adhesive tape must not extend above the spine of the scapula because the skin there is often seborrheic, especially in the midline. Nor should they be placed too far laterally, because the tape would readily become wrinkled or folded.

Hirsute skin should be carefully shaved with an electric razor. The skin should not be washed with organic solvents immediately before testing.

The test area should be free from cosmetics and ointments, and it should not have been treated previously with a topical corticosteroid for 2 weeks.

If the test patches cannot be placed on the back, they may be placed on the *outer aspects of the upper arms*. The volar surfaces of the arms and other parts of the body should be avoided, because tests at these sites may give false-negative reactions.

The adhesive strips with the test units should be placed on the back without folds, because folds prevent good occlusion. With the patient's back slightly bent, the bottom of the adhesive tape is applied first and then the tape is

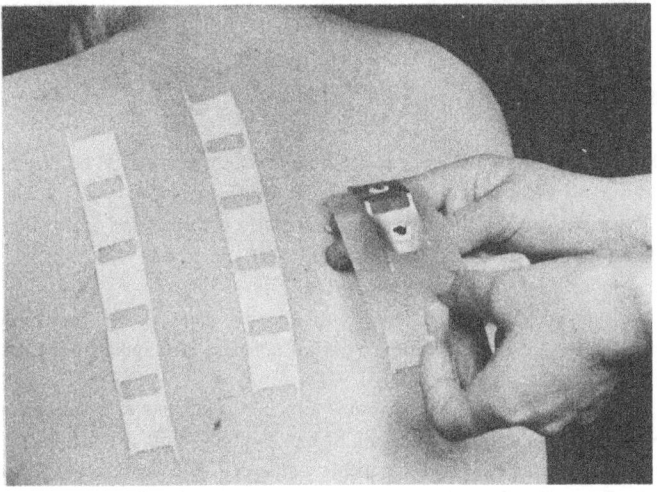

Fig. 2. Application of the test patches to the back with adhesive tape.

pressed against the skin so that the uppermost border is applied last. Then with the palm of the hand, the adhesive tape is pressed against the skin, once or twice. If the tape does not adhere well, more strips may be placed transversally over the edges of each adhesive strip. This is also advisable if the patient sweats or cannot avoid abrupt movements.

2.11 Skin Marking

Marking should always be done on the same side of the test site, lateral to the edge of the adhesive tape and preferably at the time of application. If the distance between the patches is constant, a matrix, with marks that show the site of each test, can be used. In this case, it is only necessary to mark the ends of each test row.

Ideally the marks should remain visible for a week. The following marking preparations are recommended:

1. Pyrogalol   5 g
   Ferric (III) chloride:
   saturated in water 8 ml
   Acetone   20 ml
   Ethanol   40 ml
2. Silver nitrate   50 g
   Fuchsin   2 g
   Water   75 ml
   Ethanol to give   500 ml
   To be kept in amber-colored glassware. Silver nitrate will stain clothing.
3. Dihydroxyacetone 20 g
   Water   50 ml
   Washable ink   5 ml
   Acetone to give   100 ml
   The addition of ink provides immediate color.
4. Fluorescent substances, e.g., fluorescein sodium or rose bengal, both used in ophthalmic practice. The test sites must be irradiated with UV light, e.g., Wood's light, for reading. Some test substances are fluorescent. When the markers have disappeared, inspection by UV light can sometimes facilitate orientation.
5. Fiber-tipped markers are not suitable because the marks usually disappear quickly.

2.12 Exposure Time

If an allergic contact dermatitis or allergic test reaction is to be provoked in a sensitized person, some of the allergen must be absorbed. The exposure time in the environment may vary from a few seconds, e.g., for *Primula obconica* and for poison ivy, to several days, e.g., for textiles. Occlusion by clothes, gloves, shoes, and skin folds facilitates absorption.

When applying a patch test, one should aim at *occlusion* but avoid irritation. For practical reasons, the exposure time must be the same for all substances and therefore might be unnecessarily long for some substances and too short for others. Few systematic investigations have been made of these aspects, but *an exposure time of 2 days* appears to be suitable.

One day is definitely not always adequate, and at present there is no evidence that more than 2 days is required. Variations in exposure time when tests are read at different times of the day are not significant.

2.13 Time of Reading

When the adhesive tape and the patch test are removed, the skin directly under the patches is depressed and a weak test reaction, i.e., erythema and papules, will not be visible. *Therefore the tests should not be read for at least half an hour after* the patches are removed. Because of the 2 days of occlusion, mild erythema sometimes occurs under the adhesive tape and under the test material. This may disappear within a few hours, but sometimes persists for 1 day. An allergic test reaction persists and may be more pronounced the day after the patch is removed. On the other hand, a weak irritant reaction commonly disappears within 1 day. When the first reading is taken half an hour after the test patches are removed, the results will often be questionable. *It might therefore be better to take the first reading 1 day after the patches are removed* (third day after application); the patient removes the adhesive tape and the test material. However, a disadvantage of this procedure is that one can never be sure whether the patch has become loose and must rely on the patient's report.

Because some reactions appear even later, the results should be read again on the fourth or fifth day after application, especially if the results were read for the first time 2 days after application. Of course sometimes it is necessary to vary the time of reading, e.g., when weekends intervene.

2.14 Advice to the Patient

The patient should understand the nature of the investigation. Therefore, he should be given some information. The following instructions are recommended.

In order to establish whether you are allergic to certain materials or substances, a series of patch tests has been applied to the skin on your back. These patch tests may identify the cause of an allergic dermatitis. The patch tests must *be left in place* for 2 days and 2 nights. During this time, or some days later, a red area about 10–15 mm in size may appear, which may itch. As a rule, such reactions indicate that you are allergic to the corresponding substances. In order to increase the reliability of the tests, the following precautions should be observed.

1. You should not bathe, shower, or wash your back where the patch tests are applied.
2. Avoid excessive exercise which causes heavy sweating.
3. Avoid friction or rubbing the patch tests as this may cause them to become loose.
4. Avoid scratching the areas where redness and itching appear.
5. Do not expose the test area to sun or ultraviolet lamp.

6. Should the patch test or adhesive tape become loose, apply additional adhesive tape to the patch so that it is again fixed to the original area.

   On your next visit, please tell the doctor that you had to refasten the test patch.

Removal of the Test Patches

Remove patch tests and throw away.

Date: _____

Revisit doctor: _____

   Date: _____

Appointment time: _____

7. If you observe a late reaction at the test site within 3 weeks of your visit to the doctor, you should report it.

3. Types of Reactions

3.1 Allergic Reactions

Erythema alone is not a definite sign of an allergic reaction and should usually be regarded as questionable. Certain products, however, such as cosmetics, ointments, and textiles may contain a low concentration of the allergen, and in these instances erythema alone may be a true positive reaction.

Erythema must not be confused with a reddish hue, which may be caused by certain dyes.

An allergic-type reaction not only consists of erythema but of *induration* as well, so that all reactions should be palpated. There are often *papules* and *vesicles*. Sometimes the vesicles coalesce to form small *bullae*. The reaction often extends *beyond the site of application*, especially if it is intense, but this is not a mandatory sign.

If the reaction is intense, vesicles may be seen in the actual application area and papules sometimes appear on the surrounding skin.

At times there are only papules with no erythema, e.g., positive reactions to neomycin or nickel, but by the following day the intensity of the reaction may

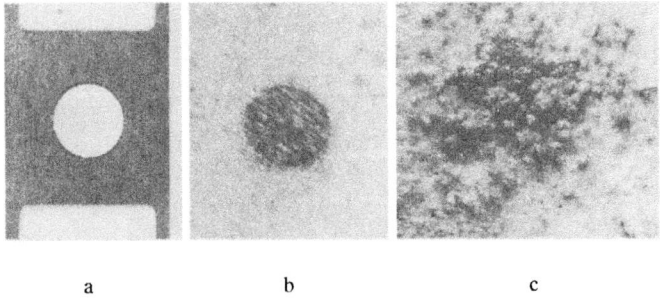

a   b   c

Fig. 3. Patch test unit and reactions (actual size). a: The filter paper is affixed at the center of a larger piece of impermeable inert material. b: The irritant reaction, with redness but without papules and vesicles, is sharply limited to the application area. c: The allergic reaction, with redness, papules and vesicles has spread beyond the application area.

20

have increased so that the erythema has coalesced and papules are seen over the entire test area.

The patient may report localized *itching* of certain test sites and there is often mild diffuse itching over the entire test area immediately after the patches are removed.

Many test reactions of an allergic type *increase in intensity the day after the patches are removed*, but they generally regress within a few days later. If it is not treated, a very intense reaction may persist for 3–4 weeks.

3.2 Late Reactions

A reaction developing 6 days or more after the patch is applied, a "late reaction," may *indicate patch-test sensitization*. It may also indicate that the existing allergic reaction has increased to such a level that residual substance on or in the skin causes a reaction. (This type of a reaction is called a "flare-up.") The absence of such a late reaction is no guarantee that test sensitization has not occurred, because these late reactions are relatively rare in patch-test-sensitized persons.

A late reaction may occur as long as 3 weeks after the test, occasionally even later. Patients who are not followed up regularly should be instructed to report any such reaction.

3.3 Irritant Reactions

There are different types of irritant reactions:

1. A *faint erythema* without infiltration, which usually disappears within 1 day after the patch is removed.
2. *Redness with a brown tinge*, often sharply outlined, which may persist for a day or so but will not become more intense.
3. Patchy *erosions,* usually without infiltration and confined to the application area. They are often caused by alkaline substances.
4. *Glazed reaction* (*effet du savon*) sharply confined to the application site; the skin is red, brownish, or a normal color with a glistening surface, and is finely wrinkled, without infiltration. This is caused by soaps, hexachlorophene, and shampoos.
5. *Bullae*, often without surrounding erythema, are sharply outlined and confined to the area of the patch. They are caused by some solvents, such as white spirit, among others. In contrast, a bullous reaction of allergic type often appears as vesicles, papules, erythema, and infiltration in the margin outside the application area.

21

Erythematous reactions may be caused by pressure from solid test material. *Pustular reactions* may develop to metals and *purpuric reactions* to *p*-phenylenediamine derivatives. Allergic reactions to phenyl-isopropyl-*p*-phenylenediamine (IPPD) may also be purpuric. *Necroses*, deeper changes which involve the dermis, leave scars. They may be caused by strong acids or alkalis and also by other chemically active substances.

It should be observed that *reactions of an irritant and allergic type may occur simultaneously*. The allergic reaction may be recognizable in the surrounding area, while the central application site contains bullae or erosions. A marginal ridge-like reaction, with papules and vesicles centrally, may suggest simultaneous allergic and irritant reactions.

Some substances, such as lower unsaturated alcohols, aldehydes, and quaternary ammonium compounds, produce irritant effects which are *clinically identical to allergic reactions*.

3.4 Irritant Reactions in Children, the Aged, and Atopic Subjects

The skin is often sensitive in children, especially those under 10; the aged with atrophic, dry skin; and atopic subjects with xerotic skin. This applies in particular to substances with test concentrations close to the irritant threshold for normal adults, such as formaldehyde, tars, quaternary ammonium compounds, detergents, cobalt, and mercury. If the test reaction to these substances is not definitely of the allergic type, the substances should be regarded as irritant. Low concentrations may be tried first in these subjects, preferably 50%–75% of the standard concentration. Often they also react to the adhesive tape.

3.5 Differentiation between Allergic and Irritant Reactions

Appearance
In many cases it is possible to distinguish clinically between the two types of reactions, but irritant responses to some substances cannot be distinguished from allergic reactions.

Chemistry
If the substance is alkaline or acid, an irritant effect may be suspected. This is also true if the test substance contains strong oxidizing or reducing agents or certain undiluted solvents, e.g., white spirit or chloroform. Organic bromo or chlor compounds have an irritant effect, even when used in low concentrations.

Reaction in Controls
If the test concentration is close (0·5–0·25) to that which causes irritant reactions in some control subjects, the reaction may also be suspected of being irritant in patients with dermatitis.

Time of Development of the Reaction
A reaction visible within a few hours is often an irritation. Reactions which do not develop until 3–5 days after the test patch unit is applied are probably not of the irritant type.

Strength of the Reaction
An extremely strong reaction to a substance that produces only a weak or no reaction in the controls is probably an allergic type.

Histology
Histologic changes in allergic reactions begin as soon as 6–8 hours after application and precede clinical signs. It can be difficult to distinguish between these different types of histologic reactions, so that biopsy is of little value in routine work.

3.6 Treatment of Test Reactions

After the last reading, test reactions can be treated with topical corticosteroids. If the reactions are multiple or intense, or if the adhesive tape has caused a severe allergic reaction, systemic treatment with corticosteroids for a few days should be considered.

3.7 Recording the Reactions

The patient's records should include a printed patch test form listing the standard series, with space for additional test substances; the vehicle and concentration should be noted for each substance. The time the tests are applied, when they are removed, and the days on which the results were read should be recorded. The positions of the tests on the body should be illustrated in a diagram.

Since differences caused by applications of the tests at different times of the day are unimportant, the time after application should be given in days, e.g., D2, D3, D5 (D — days after application). Reactions developing on D6 or later are regarded as late reactions, i.e., possible test sensitization.

The intensity of the reaction to any substance depends not only on the immunologic state of the patient and skin permeability, but also on several external factors, such as concentration, vehicle, test material, adhesive tape, season, temperature, and humidity. Testing on several different occasions may therefore give different results, although the patient's allergy remains unchanged. The intensity of the actual test reaction is not very important and should not be graded according to a too-detailed scale.

Various classifications of test reactions have been suggested. The following classification is recommended:

? +   *Doubtful reaction:* faint erythema only.
  +   Weak (nonvesicular) positive reaction; erythema, infiltration, possibly papules.
  + +   *Strong* (vesicular) positive reaction; erythema, infiltration, papules, vesicles.
+ + +   *Extreme* positive reaction; bullous reaction
  ··   *Negative* reaction.
  IR   *Irritant* reactions of different types
  NT   *Not tested.*

3.8 False-Negative Reactions

A false-negative reaction means that patch testing has failed to provoke a positive reaction despite the presence of contact allergy. Failure to react can, of course, be due to the fact that the patient had not been tested with the correct sensitizer, probably because it was not included in the standard series or the patient's history was incomplete.

A false-negative reaction in the true sense of the term is said to be present if an allergic patient does not react positively to the patch test performed with the proper sensitizer.

False-negative reactions may be caused by several factors.

Allergy State
If the tests are carried out shortly after the eczema has subsided, the state of allergy may have decreased.

If the strength of the allergy is below the threshold of the test substance applied in the usual concentration, in the technique used, the reaction will be negative. On clinical exposure, however, irritants acting simultaneously may increase the permeability of the skin to such an extent that an allergic reaction is elicited.

Concentration of Test Substance
The concentration of the test substance may be low, especially in the case of substances not belonging to a standard series. Products such as cosmetics, drugs, textiles, leather, and rubber often contain a concentration of the sen-

sitizer too low to elicit a positive reaction with the patch test on normal skin, although it is sufficient to provoke such a reaction on clinical exposure. Other products must be diluted in order to lower the concentration of their irritant components, e.g., cutting oils, soaps, detergents, glues. In such cases it is necessary to test the ingredients separately or, possibly, extracts of the products should be neutralized rather than diluted.

Amount of Test Substance
The reaction is liable to be false-negative if the volume of the solution containing the test substance is so low that the patch is not properly saturated.

Wrong Composition of Test Substance
Turpentine must be oxidized because the peroxides of delta-3-carene and other terpenes are allergens. The composition of balsams, tars and other mixtures with unknown sensitizers may differ. The content of cosmetics, household preparations, and technical preparations may have changed during their storage at testing laboratories or may have been altered by the manufacturers so that the patient is not tested with the same formulation as that to which he had previously been exposed.

Long storage may result in decomposition or polymerization, chemically altering substances, e.g., certain plastics (acrylic and carbamide).

Vehicle
The vehicle must release the test substance so that it can penetrate into the skin. Some ointment bases do not have this property. The test substance must be finely divided in the vehicle. Test preparations in petrolatum often give more reliable positive reactions than do corresponding solutions.

Occlusion
Comparative studies have shown that total occlusion decreases false-negative reactions. Such occlusion can be achieved by using an impermeable sheet and nonporous tape with good adhesive properties. The occlusion is facilitated further if petrolatum is used as the vehicle. Incomplete occlusion may occur during actual application, if the patch is put on in such a way as to produce a skin fold or if it becomes detached.

Test Site
If sites other than the back or outer surface of the upper arm are used, e.g., inner surface of the arm, a false-negative reaction may result.

Reading
If the test reaction is read immediately after the test material has been removed, the reaction may be negative, especially if the patch has adhered so

well as to cause a slight depression in the skin. A reaction may also occur later, up to the day 6 after application.

Local Corticosteroids
If tests are performed with ointments containing corticosteroids, a negative reaction may be the result for, e.g., lanolin, preservatives, antibacterial and antifungal agents, especially when these substances are present in low concentration.

Systemic Corticosteroids
Large doses of systemic corticosteroids may prevent the development of a reaction. As a rule, prednisone in doses up to 20 mg does not involve this risks.

Photosensitization
If there is only photosensitivity to a substance, the reaction may not occur without UV irradiation.

Cytostatic agents can depress a delayed reaction and a patient may show a negative patch test reaction to a topically applied pharmaceutical preparation that previously caused an allergic contact dermatitis.

3.9 False-Positive Reactions

A false-positive reaction implies that the test response seems positive in the absence of contact allergy. This means that these reactions are an irritant type. However, even an experienced investigator may sometimes be unable to decide whether a reaction is an allergic or irritant type (see Chap. 3.5). Furthermore, a misleading allergic reaction may develop if the test unit contains a sensitizer, e.g., glue, antioxidant, or plasticizer, to which the patient is sensitive.

Most substances used for patch testing may cause an irritant reaction, if they are allowed to act on the skin long enough in sufficiently high concentration.

Reliable methods are available for determining the irritant capacity of the substance.

The concentration of allergen must be adjusted according to its irritating capacity.

The ability of individuals to give an irritant reaction varies widely and some subjects will even give irritant responses to substances at the standardized test concentration. However, in most cases it is substances which the patient has brought from his environment for testing that cause these irritant reactions.

There are several causes of irritant reactions.

  1. The concentration of the actual test substance used was *too high*. This can also result from evaporation during storage.

2. The test substance is *contaminated* by an irritant.
3. The *vehicle* is irritant.
4. The *amount of test substance* in the solution applied to the patch was too large, causing overflow.
5. The test was applied on an *irritable site*, e.g., upper part of the back or trunk.
6. The existing dermatitis is in an *acute stage* or is very widespread.
7. *Dermatitis near the test site.*
8. The test site was *recently dermatitic.*
9. A strong reaction to the adhesive tape may cause a false-positive reaction to some test substances.
10. The test unit was applied to an area of the skin on which *a test had been applied before.*
11. The patient has a *very sensitive skin*, but no eczema.
12. The reaction was *read* too early after the patch was removed, e.g., after a few hours, when there was mild erythema which had disappeared by the following day.

False-negative reactions	False-positive reactions
Level of sensitivity is low	Concentration too-high for the patient in question
Test concentration is too low	The vehicle has evaporated during storage
Amount of test substance is too small	Test substance is contaminated by an irritant
Test substance is of the wrong composition	The vehicle is an irritant
Vehicle does not release the test substances	Too much of the test substance has been applied
Occlusion is insufficient	Application to the wrong anatomic site
Test site is in the wrong anatomic area	Dermatitis in an acute phase
Reading taken too early	Dermatitis near the test site
Local corticosteroid depresses the reaction	Test site has recently been dermatitic
Systemic corticosteroid depresses the reaction	Test site has recently been used for patch testing
Testing in a refractory phase	Pressure effect of solid material
Cytostatic agent depresses the reaction	Patient has an irritable skin
No UV irradiation in photosensitivity	Reading is taken too early and the reaction misinterpreted
	Intense reaction to the adhesive tape

4. Other Test Methods

4.1 Open Test

In the open test, absorption is not increased by occlusion. In cases with a high degree of allergy, a sufficient amount of the allergen can be absorbed, even if the concentration applied is the same as that used for the closed patch test. The absorption of certain substances may be less dependent on occlusion. Primin (Isolan) produces an equally strong reaction with the open test as with the closed patch test.

The test substance should be dissolved in a volatile solvent, such as acetone, alcohol, or butylacetate. Solvents that produce an irritant reaction in the closed patch test may also be used safely. Cosmetics or topical pharmaceutical preparations may be applied as sold.

The test solution is dropped onto the skin and is allowed to spread by itself over a surface, varying with the nature of the solvent. After the solution evaporates, the skin is covered only by ordinary garments. The substance may be applied *to the patient's back* or to the *outer surface of the upper arm,* as in the closed patch test.

The results are read like those of the closed patch test, but the development of the reaction can readily be followed throughout its course. Initially, there may be only erythema or isolated papules.

In very sensitive persons, several substances may produce a positive reaction, but a negative reaction does not exclude a medium degree of sensitivity with the same certainty as does a closed patch test. Substances such as primin and the catechols in poison ivy are readily absorbed, producing reactions when used in concentrations commonly used for closed patch tests.

A positive open-test reaction can usually be regarded as a sign of allergy, but some substances may also cause an irritant effect when applied in this way. Thus, organic chloro- and bromo- compounds (Mace, etc.) produce an irritant vesicular reaction, which is easily confused with an allergic response.

The open test can be recommended above all when a *high degree of sensitivity is suspected and for unknown substances.* If the reaction is negative, the test can then be supplemented with the closed patch test.

4.2 Intracutaneous Test

Intracutaneous testing has been recommended for certain contact sensitizers which are not always absorbed in sufficient amounts to give a positive reaction when applied epicutaneously, e.g., neomycin, gentian violet, Merthiolate, Rivanol, Salvarsan, ragweed oleoresin, and penicillin.

As a rule, concentrations for intracutaneous tests are one-tenth to one-hundredth those used in the patch test. Salts of chromium, cobalt, and nickel, injected in solutions of 1 mM in saline, produce reactions comparable to those obtained in patch tests with the standard concentration.

Patients are injected intracutaneously with 0·1 ml of the sterile test solution. The reaction is read 2–3 days after the injection. An erythematous papule at least 5 mm in diameter is considered a positive response.

If the proper technique for patch testing is used, there is rarely any clinical indication for intracutaneous testing, except in research work.

4.3 Testing on Mucous Membranes

Sensitizers that cause allergic stomatitis usually produce positive reactions on the skin, whereas reactions on the buccal mucosa occur more readily than those on the skin. Tests on the oral mucosa are therefore rarely indicated.

The test can be performed in the following way. The suspected substance or product is incorporated in Orabase®, an adherent paste consisting of pectin, gelatin, sodium carboxymethyl cellulose, and plasticized hydrocarbon gel. The inner side of the lip is dried, and Orabase containing the test substance is applied.

The test is read 1 and 2 days after application. Erythema and small vesicles suggest a positive reaction.

5. Photo Patch Testing

5.1 Principle

The photoallergic reaction is equivalent to the contact allergic reaction and the phototoxic reaction equivalent to the irritant (also known as "toxic") reaction.

Before photo patch-testing—or at the same time—the following should be established by photo testing: the MED read after 1 day (wavelength < 320 nm) is normal, the MED causes only erythema, long-wave UV light (> 320 nm) does not elicit skin reaction.

5.2 Source of Light

The ideal light source is the sun, but for practical reasons in many countries, artificial light sources must be used. These should have a continuous light spectrum. A carbon arc is impractical. Xenon lamps are expensive but suitable for research. Mercury·quartz lamps give a discontinuous spectrum. A variation of these, the Kromayer lamp, can be used in clinical practice. Wood's light can also be used.

For practical use, *fluorescent tubes* are recommended. They are relatively inexpensive, give off both short- and long-wave UV light continuously, have a relatively constant emission, and cover large exposure areas. When window glass is used as a filter, only long-wave (> 320 nm) light is obtained. This source of light can also be used for photo testing.

The source consists of four fluorescent lamps (24-in. tubes); two with short-wave UV light and two with long-wave:

Sunlamps: (280 nm–355 nm; max 310 nm)
  Westinghouse Sunlamp FS 20 T12
Blacklights: (320 nm–440 nm; max 350 nm)
  Westinghouse F20 T12 BLB
  General Electric F20 T12 BLB
  Osram L 20W/73

The two different types of tubes are mounted alternately, 25 mm from each other, in a box with a 15 × 30-cm opening that can be protected with window glass 2 mm thick. This opening should be 25 cm from the tubes. Behind them, there should be a light-reflecting aluminium plate.

The box may be hung on the wall and the patient may sit with the skin exposed in front of it. Alternatively, and more conveniently, the patient lies prone on a table under the box, which can be adjusted in the vertical plane.

To irradiate the photo patch test, only UV light with a wavelength of more than 320 nm, obtained by filtration through window glass, is used. This light produces no reaction on normal skin, so that it is not necessary to screen off the light from areas not tested.

Sufficient irradiation of the photo patch test with filtered light takes about 20 minutes. The actual optimal period must be calculated separately for each type of equipment.

5.3 Technique (See Scheme)

Two identical closed patch-tests, using the same test substance, are applied simultaneously and both are adequately covered with black paper. One of the patches is removed after 1 day, and before irradiation, all excess substance should be removed by washing with a suitable solvent so that the test substance does not act as a sunscreen on the skin surface.

The test site is irradiated with long-wave UV light. The results are read after a further day. At the same time, the second test (plain patch-test) is removed and if the reaction is negative, the area is immediately covered with nontransparent material, e.g., black paper, to protect it from light. The results are read after a further 1–2 days (see scheme).

Positive photo-patch test reactions resemble plain patch test responses. Photoallergic and contact-allergic reactions to the same test substance can occur simultaneously.

If photoallergy to a drug given systemically is suspected, the therapeutic dose may be given for 2 days before irradition. A 1–2 cm² area bordered by black nontransparent paper should then be irradiated. The results are read after a further two days.

The photo patch-test reactions are recorded in the same way as plain test reactions: see Chap. 3.7.

Ph?¹	*doubtful* reaction
Ph⁺	*slight* reaction
Ph⁺⁺	*intense* reaction
Ph⁺⁺⁺	*extreme* reaction
Ph⁻	*negative* reaction
Ph T	*phototoxic* reaction
Ph NT	*not* photo patch tested

Scheme for photo patch-testing

	D0	D1	D2	D3–5
PHOTO PATCH-TEST	Test application	Removal, Irradiation	Reading[a]	Reading
PLAIN PATCH-TEST	Test application under non-transparent material	—	Removal, Reading[b], If negative, application of nontransparent material	

D: Day
[a] A positive reaction indicates photosensitivity, contact sensitivity, or both.
[b] A positive reaction indicates contact sensitivity.
[a] A positive reaction and [b] a negative reaction indicates photosensitivity.

Photosensitizers	Test conc.	Vehicle
p-Aminobenzoates	5	Petrolatum
Bithionol	1	Petrolatum
4-Chloro-2-hydroxybenzoic acid butylamide (Jadit)	5	Alcohol
Chlorpromazine	0.1	Petrolatum
Eosin	50	Petrolatum
Fluorescein	10	Petrolatum
Halogenated salicylanilides	1	Petrolatum or acetone
Hexachlorophene	1	Petrolatum
Phenothiazines	1	Petrolatum or water
Quinine	1	Water
Rivanol (diaminoethoxyacridine)	2	Petrolatum

5.4 Indications

Photo patch testing should preferably be limited to those patients whose *dermatitis raises suspicion of photoallergic contact dermatitis*.

Photocontact dermatitis usually has a characteristic clinical pattern, except when it is localized exclusively on the dorsa of the hands.

Phototoxic reactions, for example those due to plants, are not an indication for photo patch-testing.

If after marketing one particular substance has caused a considerable number of cases of photo-allergic contact dermatitis, routine testing with it may be performed. Suspected photoallergic contact dermatitis due to a cosmetic product in which ingredients are unknown may indicate testing with a selected series of photosensitizers, e.g., hexachlorophene, bithionol, dichlorophene, and halogenated salicylanilides.

6. Patch Test Results Used in Clinical Management

6.1 Interpretation of Reactions

A true positive allergic test reaction indicates that the person tested has been exposed to and has thereby become sensitized to the test allergen. The test substance may be a single chemical, or the response may be to one chemical in a test mixture, or it may be a cross-reaction. It is not necessary for the patient to have, at that time, or to have had dermatitis previously caused by exposure to the substance in question.

The reaction may be *expected* and is then easy to explain (confirming test reaction).

Some *unexpected* reactions to substances in the standard series may be explained by *renewed inquiry into the patient's history* or possibly by examination of the patient's environment, e.g., place of work (informative test reaction).

The following points should be considered when explaining the significance of the reactions.

Reaction Explained by the Actual Dermatitis
Judging from the patient's history and the site of the dermatitis, contact with the substance in question has occurred in relation to the present episode of dermatitis.

Reaction Explained by Previous Episode of Dermatitis
The test substance in question has caused previous dermatitis but does not explain the present episode.

6.2 Inexplicable Reactions

The reasons why no explanation can be found may be one or more of the following.
1. *Lack of knowledge* on the part of the examiner.
2. Some sources of the substance in question *have not been traced.*
3. The patient has *not given sufficient information*, perhaps partly because the examiner did not ask the right questions.

4. The substance *occurs widely* in every environment so that a significant contact cannot be established by reference to the patient's history. Such substances are nickel, chromium, cobalt, formaldehyde, colophony, balsams, tars.
5. The patient has never developed dermatitis from the substance as he has *not been exposed to sufficient amounts* since sensitization.
6. Contact has occurred only with a *cross-reacting substance*, which may have a quite different use. If the substance is not chemically defined and occurs widely, it is difficult to trace the sensitizing exposure.

6.3 Definite Diagnosis

When the results of the tests are read, all information obtained from the patient's history, examination, evidence of exposure, examination of the working place, and chemical analyses should be considered in attempts to trace the cause of the dermatitis. Negative test reactions to contactants, named in the patient's history as current, should be considered.

The reliability of the patient's information should also be estimated. Thus, the patient may have rejected suspected contactants. It is important to try to assess alternative effects of irritants and sensitizers, especially when the lesions are confined to the hands.

Differentiation from irritant dermatitis can be facilitated by the patch test, but it should be borne in mind that *negative test reactions do not exclude allergic dermatitis. An irritant test reaction is of no diagnostic value.* It should also be remembered that irritant and allergic contact dermatitis may occur simultaneously, mainly on the hands and lower arms. If the test reaction is positive, the condition may be differentiated from other forms of eczema, such as atopic or seborrhea dermatitis, but it should be emphasized that allergic contact dermatitis may be secondary in a person with a constitutional eczema.

6.4 Treatment

The ultimate purpose of patch testing is to increase the information about the patient, making it possible to give as adequate therapy as possible, i.e., to avoid contact with the allergen(s). Patients must be warned not only against the product which has actually caused the dermatitis but also against other products containing the same allergen, or cross-reacting substances or both. It is often desirable to give the patients written lists of the allergens to which they are sensitive and ways of eliminating them.

6.5 Allergy Card

It would be useful if allergy cards were issued to allergic patients, especially those allergic to pharmaceutical preparations.

6.6 Prognosis

Evaluation of the prognosis of contact dermatitis is necessary, medically as well as for purposes of treatment and rehabilitation. Some types of allergic contact dermatitis, e.g., those due to chromium and nickel, often have a chronic or recurrent course. Local treatment may need to be adjusted or modified, because it may have to be continued for years (avoidance of sensitizers and highly potent corticosteroids). The patient should also be informed how he can best "live with his disease."

6.7 Rehabilitation

If the contact allergen is known, it must be decided whether or not the patient can continue with his usual occupation. Proper rehabilitation places rigorous demands on the physician's knowledge of the chemical environments at various working places.

6.8 Prevention

The presence of fairly strong sensitizers at a place of work can sometimes be traced by patch testing. Preventive measures should then be taken for all employees.

6.9 Legal Aspects

Proof of a connection between a person's occupation and his dermatitis is obviously much stronger if the patient has a positive test reaction to an allergen to which he is exposed at work than if the test reaction cannot be explained or is negative.

6.10 Disadvantages of Patch Testing

The greatest disadvantage of the patch test is *the risk of patch-test sensitization* or of *raising the level of sensitivity*. Sensitization may become manifest as a "late reaction" (also called flare-up). Such late reactions are rare and the frequency of test sensitization can only be assessed by retesting, which involves a further risk.

Certain substances have a high capacity to sensitize with patch testing or to raise the allergy level, e.g., *Primula obconica* (primin), PPDA, azo compounds, poison ivy. The practical consequences of patch-test sensitization have not been properly assessed. Clinical disease after test sensitization is rare. Photo patch testing also involves the risk of sensitization.

Clinical symptoms, such as *itching*, whether from allergic or irritant reactions, usually cause only minor inconvenience. Certain reactions can cause secondary *depigmentation*, however, and photo test reactions sometimes result in *pigmentation*. Women, especially, may find the reactions unpleasant from a cosmetic point of view.

7. General Aspects of Sensitizers

7.1 A Characterization of Eczematogenic Substances as Test Reagents

There are some sensitizers which rarely irritate the skin at any concentration. Such chemicals include benzocaine, lanolin, alcohols, and neomycin. It is possible for these chemicals to sensitize without causing irritation.

Other chemicals irritate in higher concentration or under specific conditions, such as extended exposure, occlusion, or increased penetration. In this case, it is important to dilute the test ointment or solution appropriately and to follow the recommendations concerning the technique of testing. Optionally irritant chemicals include potassium dichromate, cobalt chloride, nickel sulfate, and turpentine.

In addition to this classification, eczematogenic substances can also be grouped by the following aspects.

1. Chemically defined substances (for the moment regardless of the degree of chemical purity)
2. Natural mixtures
3. Artificial mixtures

The definition of the actual allergen is difficult and hardly ever of any practical interest when a contact allergy to natural mixtures has been discovered. Thus it is important for physician and patient to know about the presence of a contact allergy, e.g., to balsam of Peru, but it is not critical to know which of the many components is responsible for the allergy.

This is not true with reactions to artificial mixtures, such as common commercial ointments or test mixtures. Thus, in a commercial preparation containing corticosteroids and neomycin, the contact allergy can be a reaction to the neomycin, the lanolin alcohols, or the parabens used as preservatives. In cases of this sort it is important to identify the substance responsible.

The reactions to standard tests (Table 3) performed at the same time often yield information important for the analysis of the reaction to the commercial preparation. Occasionally, however, it is important to inquire what substances are contained in the particular preparation and to test these.

7.2 Mixtures of Test Substances

A number of test substance mixtures are available in the form of commercial test ointments (Table 2). It is important to ensure that the substances do not interact to create new, unknown substances. The test concentration of each individual substance must be sufficient to elicit an allergic reaction without irritation.

There are several reasons why it is advisable to test these mixtures. The preservatives contained in numerous preparations marketed by the cosmetic industry and, in some countries, by the pharmaceutical industry are not identified on the container. Because the preservatives used in such preparations are often esters of *p*-hydroxybenzoic acid, the inclusion of a mixture of these esters in the test can lead to a full explanation of contact allergy. It is not important to determine which specific ester is the responsible allergen, since they often interact to cause group allergies.

The multitude of allergenic rubber chemicals leads us to test them in groups, since it would require too much effort to test each substance individually. The detailed analysis of reactions to rubber chemicals is only necessary in specific cases, for example, for legal or research purposes. On the other hand, it is useful to test individual substances in the Caine mixture and in the Medi mix because of their varied nature.

7.3 Cross-Allergy

It is not uncommon for patients to react in the same way to numerous chemically related substances. The patient is originally sensitized by one such substance and upon later exposure is unable to distinguish between the sensitizer originally responsible and other related substances with a similar chemical structure. The technical and pharmacologic nature of these chemically related substances can be completely different. For example, the sensitizing substance can be a dye stuff, and the triggering substance a local anesthetic, or a preservative in an ointment. Such substances form a group. The nosologic process described above is termed a cross-allergy. Several cross-allergy groups have been described, for example the para group substances (Table 5), the derivatives of hydroxyquinoline, and the antibiotics related to neomycin. The cross-allergy can be viewed as sensitization to an allergen core common to all of these substances. In the case of a reaction of this kind, it is wise to inform the patient of the importance of cross-reacting substances.

7.4 Concomitant Allergy

It can often be observed that several substances elicit reactions in the same patient, although they are not chemically related. Reactions of this kind have their origin in the fact that they occur together during exposure. In patients with dermatitis of the lower-leg, expositional bundling can be caused by medications containing the potent allergens neomycin, lanolin, and parabens in the same commercial preparation. They can also be produced by being combined in one occupational substance, for example, chromate and cobalt in cement.

7.5 Standard Tests

The standard test substances in Table 3, chosen according to the studies of the ICDRG, are of particular importance with respect to the epidemiology of contact dermatitis. They can be ordered from Trolab as test ointments in petrolatum (Petrolatum Ph. Nord. 63). Only turpentine oxide and formaldehyde are diluted with olive oil and water, respectively. The test substances are arranged on the patient's back in three rows, with six patches each. They must be so arranged that substances which might react simultaneously because of a group or concomitant allergy are not next to each other vertically or horizontally. In this way, the direct potentiation of possible reactions which might disturb the reading of the reactions is minimized. The individual substances contained in the recommended standard test kit are detailed in Chap. 8. It can be useful to supplement the standard test with other substances or to modify it according to the region in which it is performed.

8. Special Aspects of Sensitizers[1]

8.1 Chinoform = 5-chloro-7-iodo-8-quinolinol chlorquinaldol*

Hydroxyquinoline derivatives

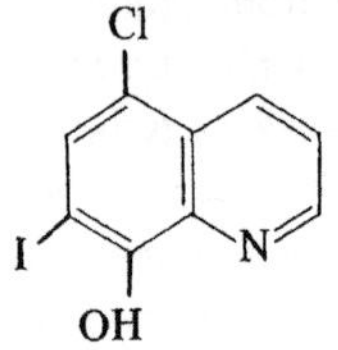

Chinoform

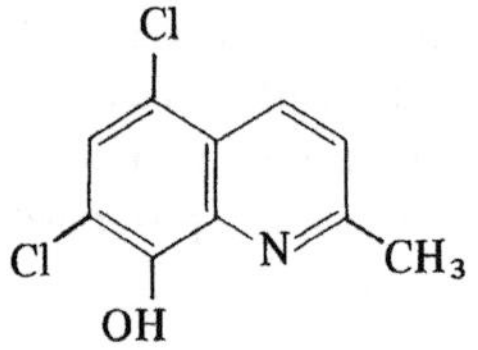

Chlorquinaldol
5,7 dichloro-2-methyl-
8-quinolinol

Iodine chloride hydroxyquinoline and chlorquinaldol are antimicrobial agents added to topical pharmaceutical preparations, including external preparations containing corticosteroids. Derivatives of hydroxyquinoline are also used as disinfectants for the pharynx (lozenges, mouthwashes, and gargles), the intestinal tract, the vulvovaginal region, and wound cavities. Some compounds are used to disinfect the hands and floors and to preserve sera and tobacco.

Sensitization occurs more frequently in countries where the substances are applied to the diseased skin in ointments or creams than in those where it is incorporated into pastes and lotions.

It is especially necessary to test this group of substances in patients who suffer from dermatitis of the lower leg or foot. Cross-reactions of the derivatives of hydroxyquinoline with each other can be observed, for example, with oxine potassium sulfate (recommended test concentration 1% in vaseline) or with 5-

---

[1] All preparations followed by an asterisk (*), in the following pages, are available as test preparations in normal commercial usage.

chlorine-8-hydroxyquinoline (recommended test concentration 1% in petrolatum).

Test concentration: iodine chlorine hydroxyquinoline 5%
                            chlorquinaldol 5%
Test vehicle: petrolatum

8.2 Chlorpromazine* Promethazine

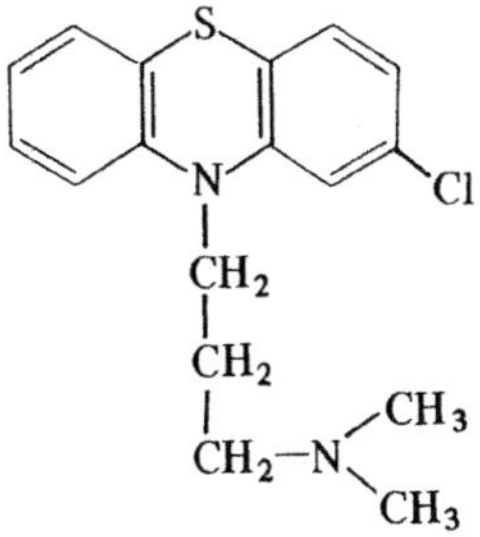

Chlorpromazine

2-Chloro-10-(3-dimethylaminopropyl)phenothiazine

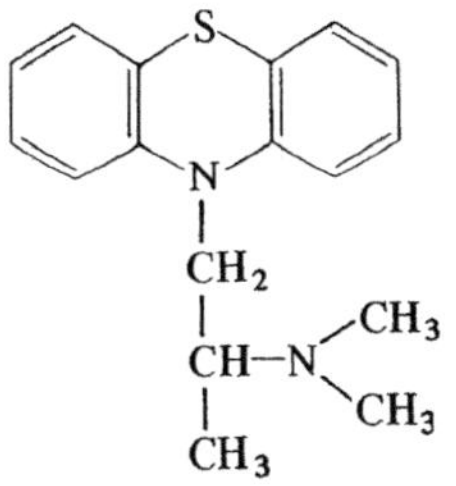

Promethazine

10-(2-Dimethylaminopropyl)phenothiazine

The chemically related phenothiazine compounds have various pharmacologic effects and are used as antiallergic agents, psychosedatives, spasmolytic agents, antiepileptic agents, parasympatholytic drugs, antiemetics, muscle relaxants, sedatives, ataractics, neuroleptic agents, and anthelmintics. Some compounds are present in insecticides and constitute an occupational hazard for gardeners and farmers. Other derivatives are added to motor oils or synthetic oils. Many dyes are phenothiazines, including methylene blue. Little is known about their sensitizing effect. They are not only contact allergens, but photoallergens as well.

Promethazine and chlorpromazine have become known as contact allergens. Promethazine is used as an antipruritic agent in external medication. In some countries, it is one of the most commonly observed contact and photoallergens.

Along with chlorpromazine, it occasionally becomes an occupational hazard for members of the medical and nursing profession in the form of ampule solutions, suppositories, syrups, and tablets. Occupational eczemas caused by phenothiazine derivatives, which occur as intermediate products, can have a sensitizing effect on the latter. Cross-reactions of phenothiazine derivatives with each other are sometimes observed.

Test concentration: Promethazine (hydrochloride) 0·1%
                          Chlorpromazine (hydrochloride) 0·1%
Test vehicle: Petrolatum

8.3 Epoxy Resin*

This widespread plastic (Table 6) is usually a product of the condensation of epichlorohydrin and dioxydiphenylmethane (bisphenol A).

Table 6.   Epoxy resins in industrial work

Electric insulation
Glass wool castings
Laminators for metals
Flooring
Fillers for cracks in cement
Glue for metals, rubber, polyester resins, glass, and ceramics
Metal finish
Antirust paint

A large number of catalysts, hardeners, softeners, and bulkage materials, the potency of which, as allergens, is, in part, still unknown, make it difficult to analyze a contact allergy elicited by epoxy resins (Table 7). Allergies of this

Table 7.   Epoxy resin hardeners (curing agents)

Type	Hardener	Test concentration %	Vehicle
Aliphatic amine	Ethylenediamine		
Aliphatic amine	Diethylenetriamine (DTA)		
Aliphatic amine	Triethylenetetramine (TTA)	1·0	Water, acetone, or petrolatum
Aliphatic amine	Dipropylenetriamine		
Aliphatic amine	Dimethylaminopropylamine		
Aromatic amine	p,p-Diaminodiphenylmethane	1·0	
Acid anhydride	Phthalic anhydride	1·0	

kind are found mainly among workers in industries that use uncured epoxy resins.

In cases where such a contact allergy is suspected, it is useful to test the chemicals used by the patient.

It is important to regulate the test concentrations carefully when testing the chemicals actually used by the patient (1,2,5,12).

8.4 Benzocaine*

$$H_2N-\langle O \rangle-COO-CH_2-CH_3 \qquad \text{Ethoform}$$

4-aminobenzoic acid ethyl ester

Because of its widespread use as a surface anesthetic, test reactions produced by benzocaine are observed in approximately 4% of patients with dermatitis. Approximately 60% of the reactions can be explained.

It is used in concentrations of 0.2%–20% in burn ointments, analgesic and antiprurient ointments, dusting powders, depilatory creams, protective sun creams, shaving creams, aftershave lotions, and denture adhesives. It can also occur in sugar-coated tablets, lozenges, and wafers for the treatment of nausea, coughs, sore throat and laryngalgia. Occasionally it is used to combat motion sickness in small animals. Benzocaine should be tested, especially in patients who suffer from stasis or anal eczema.

Cross allergy:	Para group substances, sulfamylon (Table 5)
Concomitant allergy:	Lanolin alcohols, neomycin group
Test concentration:	5%
Test vehicle:	Petrolatum

8.5 Formaldehyde*

Formaldehyde is used as a disinfectant and preservative for numerous purposes. It serves as the basis for plastics, adhesives, and glues. In dermatologic therapy and cosmetics it is used as an antiperspirant. Leather tanned with formaldehyde can function as an allergen, producing foot eczemas (Table 8.

Test concentration:	2% of formaldehyde (Formalin contains about 38% formaldehyde)
Test vehicle:	Water

Table 8. Commodities and occupational products containing formaldehyde

Antifungal disinfectants
Disinfectants (in ointments, powders, lotions, washes, instruments, seed corn)
Preservatives (adhesives, cutting solution, cosmetics, tetanus serum)
Protective substances for plants, insecticides (fungicides, germicides)
Antiperspirants (powders, solutions, ointments, sticks, and inner soles for shoes)
Coal and wood smoke
Glue for the outer leaves of cigars
Leather-tanning substances
Basic material for textile finishes
Component of many varied plastics
Glue
Photographic materials (paper, plates, fixing baths)
Additives for motor oils
Fixing and preserving solution for histologic and anatomic preparations

Formaldehyde can be released from:
hexamethylene tetramine
(Urotropin)
paraformaldehyde
tricresol formaldehyde

8.6 Rubber Chemicals

Contact allergy due to rubber products is common and is an occupational hazard to workers in rubber producing and processing industries. Localization of the contact dermatitis sometimes suggests the rubber contact that produced it (Table 9a). It must also be remembered that technical rubber articles, such as tires, conveyor belts, or hard rubber (pipe mouth pieces, fountain pens) trigger the reaction. It is not the rubber itself, but the numerous chemicals used in its production or processing that are allergens.

Below is a list of the rubber chemicals most often suspected of acting as sensitizers (Table 9b). TMTD is also used as a disinfectant in scabies medication and in antimycotic agents and skin sprays. It also acts as a preservative for

Table 9a. Site of dermatitis and triggering rubber objects

Site of dermatitis	Rubber object
Finger	Rubber finger protectors, rubber erasers
Hand and wrist	Rubber gloves
Foot and lower leg	Rubber boots
Leg	Elastic bandages
Waist	Elastic bands
Genitalia	Condom
Behind the ear lobe, temples	Rubber protective glasses or mask

Table 9b. Allergenic rubber chemicals[a]

Substance	Test concentration (%)
Tetramethylthiuram disulfide (TMTD)	2
Tetramethylthiuram monosulfide (TMTM)	2
Mercaptobenzothiazole (MBT)	2
2-mercaptobenzimidazole	1
N-phenylcyclohexy-p-phenylenediamine	1
N-cyclohexyl-2-benzothiazolsulphenamide	1
N-diethyl-2-benzothiazylsulphenamide	1
Hydroquinone monobenzyl ether	1
1,3-diphenylguanidine	1
Phenyl-β-naphthylamine	1
Isopropylaminodiphenylamine	0·1
1,4-dihydroxydiphenyl	0·2
Benzoyl peroxide	1
2,2-methylene-bis(4-methyl-6-tertiary butylphenol)	1
Hexamethylenetetramine	1
Bis(diethyl dithiocarbamic acid)zinc = DDTC	1
Diphenyl-p-phenylenediamine	1
Morpholinylmercaptobenzothiazole	1
Tetraethylthiuramidisulfide	1
Dipentamethylenethiuram disulfide	1
Di-β-naphthylthiuram disulfide	1
Bis(dibutyl dithiocarbamic acid)zinc	1

[a] Vehicle: petrolatum.

wood, industrial oils, and fats and is sometimes added to cosmetics, such as suntan oils, for the same purpose. Fruits, nuts, mushrooms, and seeds are disinfected with it, and it is contained in many rose sprays. In addition to rubber articles, MBT is also found as an additive in cutting oils and as an antioxidant in plastics and synthetic fibers. Both cross-reactions of chemically related rubber chemicals and concomitant allergy are quite common.

Three test mixtures (Thiuram mix, Naphthyl mix, PPD mix, Table 2) are recommended for inclusion in a standard test to track down contact allergy to rubber chemicals (Table 3).

Table 9b lists other rubber chemicals which can be tested to analyze positive reactions to one of the above mixtures.

8.7 Chromium

The actual allergen is the chromate ion. However, trivalent chromium can also elicit a reaction, e.g., basic chromium sulfate in leather. Chromium is one of

Table 10. Occurrence of allergenic chromium

Cement
Cement adhesives
Cement plaster
Corrosion preventives in oils, fats, cutting oils
Antirust paint
Dyestuffs in blue printing dyes, glass dyes, paper dyes, lithographic dyes, paints, cement
    paints, rubber, paper bills, porcelain glazes, ink, tatoos, plastics
Fire-protective salts (impregnation for wood and frame wood for mines)
Leather and substances for the care of leather (tanning substances)
Photographic chemicals (fixing substances, developer, tinter, paper goods, color film
    developer, softener)
Laboratory chemicals (glass cleaning, histology, milk testing)
Fireworks
Match heads
Wood ash (also from matches)
Galvanized iron sheets
Delustering substances (metallurgic industry)
(Linoleum and floor wax)
Bleaches (for example Javelle's solution)
Casting molds, casting sand (heavy industry, metallurgic industry)
Bichromated gelatin (automobile fittings)
Paper flowers
Products of the chemical industry

the substances to which sensitization occurs most often, and it is found almost ubiquitously, most often in trace quantities. For this reason, patients with a contact allergy to dichromates tend to have chronically recurrent dermatitis, which can only be treated successfully when the patient is informed of the presence of this contact allergen in commodities and industrial substances. Thus, a patient suffering from a chromium contact allergy finds it difficult to locate a new job. A number of the materials listed in Table 10 also contain cobalt, and a corresponding concomitant allergy is by no means uncommon. Workers handling cement are particularly liable to chromate eczemas.

Concomitant allergy: Cobalt and nickel
Test concentration: 0.5%
Vehicle: Water or petrolatum

8.8 Cobalt

Much of what has been said about nickel is also true of cobalt. Hence, the cobalt ion must be considered to be the actual allergen. Tables 11 and 12 have almost the same validity. The frequent concomitant allergy mentioned must be stressed again here. It is especially important with respect to the fact that both

Table 11. Commodities and products containing cobalt (see also Table 12, Objects containing nickel)

Dyes in colored inks, textiles, rubber, synthetic resins, paints, water colors, chalk, glass paints, porcelain glazes, ceramic glazes, tatoos, enamel dyes, linen ink, printing dyes, fluorescent paints
Clay (pottery)
Priming (porcelain, glass, galvanization)
Galvanized objects
Corrosion protectives (oils, antifreeze)
Catalysts (chemical and pharmaceutical industries)
Animal Feed
Drying agents for varnishes and synthetic resin paints

---

cobalt salts and chromates occur in traces in cement. Allergy to cobalt salts is common.

Concomitant allergy:	Chromium and nickel
Test concentration:	1%
Vehicle:	Water or Petrolatum

8.9 Nickel

The real allergen is the nickel ion. It is one of the substances that most often elicit contact dermatitis. In addition to occupational substances, numerous commodities contain nickel (Table 12).

Table 12. Occurrence of nickel

Coins	Metal parts of shoes
Keys	Handlebars of bicycles
Doorknobs	False teeth
Water faucets	Eyeglass frames
Bathroom fittings	Fashion jewelry
Kitchen utensils	Hairclips
Vacuum cleaner	Lipstick holder
Washing machine	Underwear fasteners
Dishwasher	Zippers and garters
Sewing utensils	Instruments
Safety pins	Dial (telephone)
Writing materials	Automobile fittings
Fountain pen caps	Nickel salts (catalysts, fat refining)
Razors	Nickel alloys
Electric razors	Ceramics (paints and glazes)
Shoe horns	Artificial fertilizers (potted plants)

Table 13. Site of dermatitis and triggering objects

Site of dermatitis	Nickel object
Feet	Shoes (ornaments)
Shoulders	Adjustable fasteners for underwear
Upper legs	Garters
Wrists	Watch bands, bracelets
Finger, proximal	Rings
Finger, distal	Coins
Ear lobes	Clips
Behind the ear lobe, bridge of the nose	Spectacle frames
Neck, throat	Chains, necklaces
Mouth	Harmonica, woodwind, and brass instruments
Back	Zippers, brassiere hooks

Localization of the contact dermatitis can justify a strong suspicion as to the presence of a nickel contact dermatitis (Table 13).

The cobalt or chromate contact allergy often observed at the same time can be explained as a concomitant allergy. Many materials contain cobalt or chrome salts in addition to nickel, even if only in traces.

Concomitant allergy:	Chromium and cobalt
Test concentration:	5%
Vehicle:	Water or petrolatum

A	B
1% Dimethylglyoxime in alcoholic solution	10% Ammonium hydroxide solution

Directions: A few drops of (A) plus a few drops of (B) added to a metallic object or solution will produce a strawberry red insoluble salt in the presence of available nickel.

Identification of nickel according to A. Fisher. (Test solutions available from Westwood Pharmaceuticals, Inc., United States.)

8.10 Lanolin Alcohols*

Lanolin alcohols are obtained from anhydrous Adeps lanae. This fat, which melts at approximately 40°C, is obtained from merino wool and serves as emulsifier in many ointments or ointment-like products. Lanolin is the designation for various ointment bases composed in a number of ways but all containing quite a high percentage of lanolin alcohols.

It seems likely that a group of straight-chain aliphatic fat alcohols, not potent allergens in themselves, are the actual allergens in the various emulsifiers containing lanolin alcohol.

Their wide distribution and frequent use explain why they elicit positive test reactions in approximately 2·5% of all dermatitis patients.

Since lanolins or their purified extracts (for example Eucerin) are put together in various ways, it is not surprising that they do not always elicit concordant test reactions. For this reason, the test should be performed not only with a standard test substance, but also with the lanolin or lanolin preparation suspected.

Lanolin is a component of numerous local therapeutic agents and cosmetics, including ointments, creams, lotions, sprays, protective sun creams, hand creams, refreshing creams, day creams, cleansing creams, shampoos, hair lotions, setting lotions, shaving soaps, creams, aftershaves, toilet soaps, bath salts, and industrial protective hand creams.

It is not so well-known that the following articles are also treated with lanolin: condoms, polishes, substances for sealing metals, furniture polish, water-repellent substances, oilskins, leather boots, shoe polish, ski wax, isolating substances for cables, insect sprays, carbon paper, and cutting-oil emulsions.

Allergy to lanolin alcohols is most often detected in lower-leg dermatitis. Such lanolin contact allergy is not uncommonly associated with allergy to neomycin, balsam of Peru, parabens, antibiotics of the neomycin group, or hydroxyquinoline derivatives. It is not expedient to use test vehicles containing lanolin derivatives.

Test concentration: 30%
Test vehicle: Petrolatum

8.11 Mafenide* Sulfatolamide, Sulfamylon

$$H_2N-CH_2 \underset{\bigcirc}{} SO_2-NH_2 \qquad \text{Mafenide}$$

2-amino-p-toluenesulfonamide (hydrochloride)

$$H_2N \underset{\bigcirc}{} SO_2NH_2 . H_2N \underset{\bigcirc}{} SO_2NHCSNH_2$$

sulfatolamide
salt of Mafenide with 1-sulfanilyl-2-thiourea

Mafenide and its salt, sulfatolamide, almost always produce identical reactions on patch testing. Both of these chemical therapeutic agents, which are closely related to the sulfonamides, are used almost exclusively as topical therapeutic agents.

Whereas Mafenide, combined with sulfanilamide, is applied chiefly in the form of a powder and worked into gauze bandages, sulfatolamide is also sold as a salt suspension for instillations, and together with Cyren B and adipic acid as vaginal tablets.

In contrast to other European countries, contact allergy to Mafenide is observed relatively often in Germany.

Cross-reactions are often elicited by para-substituted aromatic amines (para group substances, Table 5) but seldom by sulfanilamides.

Test concentration: Mafenide 10%
Test vehicle: Petrolatum

8.12 Neomycin*

Neomycin A

4·6-Diamino-1(2·6-diamino-2·6-didesoxy-β-D-glucosyloxy)
−(1S : 2S : 3R : 4S : 6R)-cyclohexandiol-(2·3)

Neomycin has found widespread use as an antibiotic applied chiefly for local therapy. For this reason, in spite of its actual slight potency as an allergen, it is one of the pharmaceutical preparations that most frequently induce contact allergy, triggering test reactions in approximately 4% of all patients with dermatitis.

Neomycin is sold in various compounds which elicit practically identical reactions: Neomycin A, Neomycin B (Framycetin), Neomycin C, Neomycin sulfate, Neomycin-undecylenate, and Neomycin oleate.

Cross-reactions are frequently observed to the antibiotics kanamycin and paromycin, which are closely related chemically, but less often to gentamycin and streptomycin.

Because neomycin is not uncommonly combined with bacitracin in local therapeutic agents, concomitant allergies to this antibiotic, which is actually only a weak sensitizer, are sometimes seen.

Almost all local therapeutic forms for application contain neomycin. Its wide distribution is due especially to its function as an additive to topical agents containing corticosteroids.

Corticosteroids or antihistamines in topical pharmaceutical preparations do not prevent sensitization or dermatitis caused by neomycin or chemically related antibiotics. In special preparations, neomycin can be introduced into wounds or tooth roots. It is added to some deodorants. Neomycin contact allergy is discovered quite frequently in the case of lower-leg dermatitis.

Test concentrations that are too weak are the cause of many false-negative reactions.

Cross allergy: Kanamycin, paromycin, gentamycin, streptomycin
Concomitant allergy: Bacitracin, lanolin alcohols, Peru balsam, parabens, benzocaine

Test concentration: 20%
Test vehicle: Petrolatum

8.13 Colophony (Rosin)

It consists of various resin acids, predominantly (more than 90%) abietic acid, and is obtained from the distillation residue of raw conifer balsam, conifer roots, or tall oil. It occurs in numerous substances in daily use (Table 14). For this reason, it can be difficult to trace the cause in a given case. The colophony content in soap, for instance, is usually unknown.

Table 14. Materials containing colophony

Violin rosin
Adhesive tape
Drying agents
Filling material (soaps, rubber, plastics)
Polishes
Varnishes
Printing inks
Sealing wax
Putty
Brewery pitch
Linoleum
Water-repellent substances
Paper-refining substances
Slippage inhibitors (for clutches)
Fireworks
Grafting wax
Photographic paper
Labels

Allergic reactions due to the same allergen or a group allergy occur with: turpentine, wood tar, peru balsam, spruce and pine balsam

Test concentration: 20%
Vehicle: Petrolatum

8.14 Parabens

Due to their lack of odor and taste and their atoxicity, parabens are used as fungicide and bactericide preservatives. Their solubility is poor in water but good in alcohol and acetone.

(*p*-hydroxybenzoic acid ester)

HO—⟨benzene ring⟩—COO—R

R = —CH₃ = methyl paraben
  = methyl-*p*-hydroxybensoate

R = —CH₂—CH₃ = ethylparaben
  = ethyl-*p*-hydroxybenzoate

R = —CH₂—CH₂—CH₃ = propyl paraben
  = propyl-*p*-hydroxybenzoate

R = —CH⟨CH₃ / CH₃⟩ = isopropyl paraben
  = isopropyl *p*-hydroxybenzoate

R = —CH₂—CH₂—CH₂—CH₃ = butyl paraben
  = butyl *p*-hydroxybenzoate

R = —CH₂—⟨benzene ring⟩ = benzyl paraben
  = benzyl *p*-hydroxybenzoate

In spite of their relatively slight allergenicity, they elicit test reactions in about 2% of all patients with dermatitis because of their wide distribution. About 70% of the reactions can be explained.

If contact allergy to locally applied drugs or cosmetics is suspected, they should be tested.

The following substances can contain parabens:

1. Local therapeutic agents: tinctures, lotions, creams, ointments, corresponding mixtures for the treatment of cutaneous mucous membranes (anal, nasal, ear, and conjunctival). Methylesters and propylesters of *p*-hydroxybenzoic acid are usually added to this substance group.

2. Other medications: suppositories, antibiotics in solution to be taken orally, local anesthetics in solutions to be given by injection, cytostatic drugs in solution for injections and infusions.

3. Cosmetics, more than 50% of all preparations: preparations for skin care and toilet articles: lipstick, eye shadow, eyebrow dipilatory creams, makeup, cosmetic lotions, creams, ointments, baby ointments and pastes, deodorants, tooth pastes, tooth powder, mouth wash, shaving soaps, shaving creams, aftershaves, hair lotion, hair-setting lotion, nail polish, sunburn lotion, and suntan lotion.

4. Food: salads, canned fish, hors d'oeuvres, soda pop, fruit and vegetable juices, baked goods. (Mixtures of ethylesters and propylesters are used particularly often.)

In addition, adhesives, glues, shoe polish, and numerous other technical products that spoil easily can contain parabens.

Table 15. Niquel's test

1. $HgCl_2$ 7·0
   KNO_3 0·4
   H_2O 100·0
2. Dissolve the substances in water.
   Filter.
3. Dissolve several centigrams of the substance to be tested in alcohol.
4. Mix this solution with approximately 3 ml of the above reagent.
5. Heat the mixture in a water bath.

Result: after 10 minutes, dark red coloring appears if parabens are present.
Salicylic acid, ascorbic acid, and similar substances elicit the same color reaction.

In higher concentrations they are prescribed as antifungal agents.

Because parabens do not need to be declared in some countries, the content of the preparations common there is not known. The Niquel's test (Table 15) can be used to exclude the presence of parabens in such preparations.

Parabens can be tested as mixtures (Table 4).

Cross allergy:	Parabens among themselves
Concomitant Allergy:	Lanolin, neomycin group
Test concentration:	3%–5%
Vehicle:	Petrolatum or alcohol

8.15 Para-Dyes

(para-amino-substituted aromatic dye compounds)

(formulas see Table 5)

The compounds listed can be described together for two reasons.

1. They often lead to cross-reactions
2. They serve as indicators for dyestuff allergy, for instance to azo dyes

Such dyes are used as hair dyes (for this reason occupational noxa for hairdressers), as fur and textile dyes, as leather dyes, in rubber articles (also as antioxidants), for cosmetics (e.g., eyebrow pencil), and in shoe polish. As chemicals they are used in photography and in the synthesis of drugs and numerous chemical compounds.

Test substance	Test concentration (%)
p-Phenylenediamine[1]	1
p-Aminodiphenylamine	0·25
p-Tolylenediamine (sulfate)[1]	1
p-Aminoazobenzene	0·25
Benzidine	1

Test vehicle: petrolatum

8.16 Balsam of Peru*

It is obtained from the resin of the tree *Myroxylon pereira* (ROYLE) Klotsch, which grows in Central and South America. It is a mixture of numerous alcohols, aldehydes, acids, camphor, and other substances, some of which are unknown. Many of them can have an eczematogenic effect. The same allergens, or ones closely related chemically, are contained in a number of other balsams and essential oils. For this reason, a reaction to balsam of Peru is to be considered an indicator reaction for contact allergies to a number of spices as well as aromatic substances. Thus, the following substances can contain the compounds found in balsam of Peru or closely related ones: balsam of tolu (from the resin of *Myroxylon balsamum*), Tiger balsam, storax (*Liquidambar orientalis* Miller), spruce resin (*Picea exulsea*), pine resin (*Pinus silvetis*), the tars, birch tar (*Pix betulae*), *Pix fagis*, black pitch (*Pix liquida*), Pix cadini, gum bezoin [*Styrax tonkinense* (Pierre) Craib], citrus fruit peals, aloe, curry, myrrh, vanilla, cinnamon, colyphony, and turpentine.

Peru balsam is one of the substances that often elicit contact allergy.

This is especially true in the case of patients who suffer from lower-leg eczemas, many of which are still treated with ointments and tinctures produced as household remedies (wound and burn ointments) by small pharmaceutical firms. Some hemorrhoidal ointments, suppositories, and adhesive bandages also contain Peru balsam or tincture of benzoin. Tincture Arning, which is official in Germany (DAB 6) is mixed with this tincture.

It is difficult to trace the source of contact allergy to Peru balsam when it is hidden in aromatic substances in toilet articles, spices, food and drink, and tobacco. It is easier to identify balsams as the cause of occupational dermatitis in dentists (aromatic substance for dental cement liquids) and in porcelain painters (additive for porcelain and earthenware glazes).

Test concentration: 25%
Test vehicle: petrolatum

8.17 Mercury*, Mercury Salts*, and Phenyl-Mercury Compounds*

For epicutaneous patch testing structurally different mercury compounds can be discussed together; when tested simultaneously, they often elicit concordant reactions. The Hg^{2+} ion could be suspected as the common allergenic core. However, a number of chemical considerations which have not yet been cleared up contradict this assumption. Mercury derivatives can elicit contact allergenic reactions both as medical preparations and as occupational products. The white precipitate ointment as well as phenyl-mercury-oleate are only important today as a medication for psoriasis. The sublimate is an inexpensive, widely used disinfectant. Because of their germicidal effects, phenyl-mercury-borate and phenyl-mercury-nitrate are now used as antiseptics, fungicides, germicides, and herbicides. Thus they are components of antifungal tinctures, ointments, and gels. They are also found as spermicidally active ingredients in contraceptives. Merbromin is important as an antiseptic. Because of their disinfectant properties, mercury compounds are added to perishable drugs. They are added in low concentrations to local therapeutic agents, cosmetics (i.e., merthiolate, cialit), soaps, plasters, sera (cialit), gamma globulin, and allergenic solutions for scratch, prick, or intradermal tests.

Mercury and its compounds are used in cosmetics as bleaches for freckles or other pigmentations.

Mercurial diuretics, administered by a systemic route, occasionally elicit hematogenous contact eczemas (eczema-like drug rashes).

The disinfecting and preserving property of mercury compounds is exploited industrially. For this reason, workers who handle such products are at risk. It is found in cutting oils, seed-corn, fruits, swimming-pool paint, wood preservatives, shoe polish, floor wax, starches, and intermediate products of the paper industry.

Mercury and its compounds are also contained in denatured alcohol, tattoo stains (red), paint pigments, textile printing colors, measuring instruments, high-pressure pumps, casting molds for the manufacture of precision instruments, batteries, material for electrolytic purification of substances for nuclear fission, cathode material for galvanization, separation liquid in the metallurgic industry, catalysts in the chemical industry, photographic chemicals, currying substances for furs, fireworks, fulminating mercury, inks, leather-tanning substances, sealing substances for metals and amalgams (also for dental material).

Cross allergy: Mercury compounds among each other
Concomitant allergy: Lanolin alcohols, antimycotics of various origin

Test substance	Test concentration (%)
Merbromin*	0·2
Phenyl-mercury-borate*	0·02
Phenyl-mercury-nitrate*	0·02
Mercury*	0·5
White fusible mercury precipitate	1
Sublimate*	0·1
Merthiolate	0·1

Test vehicle: Petrolatum

8.18 Turpentine*

The composition of turpentine varies according to its origin. It is obtained chiefly from the bark and young wood of resinous conifers by various techniques.

Table 16. Drugs, cosmetics, and occupational substances containing turpentine

Chilblain ointments
Rheumatism ointments, liniments, oils, baths, and sticks
Insecticides
Adhesive bandages
Aromatic substances for soaps and bathing salts
Floor wax
Shoe polish
Sealing wax
Oil paints and varnishes
Thinners or solvents for paints and varnishes
Fat dissolver
Cutting and polishing waters or oils
Detergents for printer's rollers
Printer's ink
Green wood and sawdust of numerous evergreens

The actual sensitizers are the peroxides of Δ3-carene, α-pinene, β-pinene, and limonene.

If a turpentine allergy is suspected, not only turpentine obtained from one of the sources mentioned (Table 16) should be tested, but a dilution of the substance (5% in olive oil) actually used by the patient should also be tested.

Concomitant allergy: Colophony, wood tar, Peru balsam, spruce and pine resin
Test concentration: Turpentine peroxide 0.3%
Vehicle: Olive oil or petrolatum

9. Test Substances

Table 17a. Test substances marketed

Symbols and abbreviations:

▲	Vehicle: petrolatum Ph. Nord 63,	amount	5-ml package polypropylene syringe
▼	Vehicle: petrolatum	amount	2·5-ml package polypropylene syringe
■	Vehicle: petrolatum	amount	10·0-ml package aluminium tube
□	Vehicle: petrolatum	amount	5·0-ml package aluminium tube
●	Vehicle: water	amount	10·0-ml package glass bottle
⊙	Vehicle: olive oil	amount	10·0-ml package glass bottle
⊙	Vehicle: patch test unit (prepared)		package 5 Al-test units in aluminium foil
○	Vehicle: water	amount	3·0-ml package glass bottle
(Ph)	Photosensitizer		
(WHO)	World Health Organization		
(DAB)	German pharmacopoea		

Addresses

Hermal-Chemie Kurt Herrmann
D-2057 Reinbeck (BRD)

Hollister-Stier Laboratories
Spokane Washington (USA)
Box 3145 Term. Annex
Zip Code 94577

Dr.Friedrich Sasse
(Zweingniederlassung der Godecke Aktiengesell-
  schaft in Berlin)
D-78 Freiburg (BRD)
Postfach 1423
Trolab laboratory for dermatologic tests
Karen Trolle-Lassen, M. Pharm.
65 A.N. Hansens alle'
DK-2900 Hellerup (Denmark)

Table 17a—continued

Test substance[a]	Firm	No.	Trade name	Test concentration (%)	Vehicle, etc.
Acrylic monomer	Hollister-Stier		Acrylic Monomer	10	▼
Adeps lanae → Lanolin alcohol					
p-Aminoazobenzene	Trolab	0501	p-Aminoazobenzene	0·25	◀
p-Aminodiphenylamine	Dr. Sasse	16	p-Aminodiphenylamin	0·25	◀ ■
p-Aminodiphenylamine	Trolab	0300	p-Aminodiphenylamine	0·25	◀
p-Aminomethylbenzolsulfonamide →Mafenid					
Amethocaine → Tetracaine					
Atropine	Dr. Sasse	M37	Atropinsulfat	1	■
Benzocaine → Ethoform					
Tct. Benzoes	Hermal	22	Tinctura Benzoes	5	□
	Dr. Sasse	AM32	Tct. Benzoes	10	■ ■
Benzoyl Peroxide	Dr. Sasse	G21	Benzoylperoxyd	1	◀
	Trolab	0201	Benzoylperoxyde	1	■ ◀
Bithionol (WHO) (Ph)	Dr. Sasse	AM30	Bithionol	1	■ ◀
	Trolab	0100	Bithionol	1	◀
p-Tert. butylphenolformaldehyde resin	Trolab	0902	p-Tert. butylphenolformaldehyde resin	1	◀
Chinoform → iodochlorhydroxyquin					
Chlorquinaldol (WHO)	Trolab	0104	Chlorquinaldol	5	◀
Iodochlorhydroxyquin	Allergopharma	20	Chloriodoxychinolin	2	□
	Hollister-Stier		Vioform	3	▶
	Dr. Sasse	AM28	7-iod-5-chlor-8-oxychinolin	2	■
	Trolab	0015	Chinoform	5	◀
Chlorpromazine (WHO) (Ph)	Trolab	1202	Chlorpromazine chloride	1	◀
Chlorophenothane (DDT) (WHO)	Trolab	0703	DDT (dichlorodiphenyltrichlorethane)	1	◀
Quinine hydrochloride	Dr. Sasse	M35	Chininhydrochlorid	1	■

Test substance	Supplier	Code	Product	Conc.
Chromium → Potassium dichromate				
Cinchocaine (WHO)	Hollister-Stier	0401	Nupercaine	1
	Trolab	0200	Cinchocaine chloride	1
Cinnamon oil	Trolab	10	Cinnamon oil	0·5
Coal tar	Hermal		Steinkohlenteer	3
	Hollister-Stier		Coal tar	5
	Trolab	29	Coal tar	5
Cobalt	Hermal		Kobaltsulfat	2
	Hollister-Stier		Cobalt sulfate	2·3
	Dr. Sasse	9	Kobaltchlorid	2
	Trolab	0002	Cobalt chloride	2
Colophony	Hermal	Nr.30	Kolophonium	10
	Dr. Sasse	Nr.8	Kolophonium	10
	Trolab	Nr.0017	Colophony	20
N-Cyclohexyl-2-benzthiazolsulfenamide	Dr. Sasse	G23	N-Cyclohexyl-2-benzothiazol-sulfenamid	1
	Trolab	1000	N-Cyclohexylbenzothiazylsulfenamide (CBS)	1
Cyclomethycaine	Hollister-Stier		Surfacaine	1
	Trolab	0403	Cyclomethycaine chloride	
DDT Chlorophenotane N-Diethyl-2-benzothiazosulfenamide	Dr. Sasse	G25	N-Diethyl-2-benzothiazylsulfenamid	1
4,4'-Diaminodiphenylmethane	Trolab	0906	Diaminodiphenylmethane (epoxy curing agent)	0·5
Dibenzothiazoldisulfid (MBTS)	Trolab	1014	Dibenzothiazyl-disulfide (MBTS)	1
Dibutylphthalate	Hollister-Stier	0903	Dibutyl phthalate	5
Dichlorophen (WHO) (Ph)	Trolab	1005	Dichlorophene	0·5
4,4'-Dioxydiphenyl (DOD)	Trolab		4,4'-Dihydroxy-diphenyl (DOD)	0·2
Di-β-naphthyl-p-phenylenediamine (DBNPD)	Trolab	1018	Di-β-naphthyl-p-phenylene-diamine (DBNPD)	1
Dipentamethylenethiuramdisulfide (PTD)	Trolab	1017	Dipentamethylenethiuramdisulfide (PTD)	1
1,3-Diphenylguanidine	Dr. Sasse	G26	1,3-Diphenylguanidin	1
	Trolab	1002	1,3-Diphenylguanidine (DPG)	1

Table 17a—continued

Test substance	Firm	No.	Trade name	Test concentration (%)	Vehicle, etc.
Diphenyl-p-phenylenediamine (DPPD)	Trolab	1013	Diphenyl-p-phenylene-diamine (DPPD)	1	◀
Disperse orange 3	Trolab	0502	Disperse orange 3	1	◀
Disperse yellow 3	Trolab	0503	Disperse yellow 3	1	◀
Emulsifier	Trolab	1200	Emulsifying wax	20	◀▶
Epoxy resin	Hollister-Stier	0021	Epoxy glue resin	1	◀
	Trolab	5	Epoxy resin	1	□ ▶
Ethoform (WHO)	Hermal		Benzocain	5	■
	Hollister-Stier	15	Benzocaine	5	◀▶
	Dr. Sasse		Benzocain	5	◀▶
	Trolab	0405	Benzocaine	5	◀
Ethylenediamine	Hollister-Stier		Ethylenediamine	1	◀▶
	Trolab	0027	Ethylene diamine	1	□
2-Ethoxyethyl-methoxycinnamate	Trolab	1100	Ethoxyethyl-p-methoxy-cinnamate	5	■
Ethylparaben	Hollister-Stier		Paraben, ethyl	3	◀
Eucerinum anhydricum	Hermal	3	Eucerin, anhydricum	100	◀
	Dr. Sasse	11	Eucerin, anhydricum	100	□
C.D.2. Color developer	Trolab	0803	(C.D.2. color developer)	1	○
C.D.3. Color developer	Trolab	0804	(C.D.3. color developer)	1	■
Formaldehyde	Hermal	11	Formalin	1–2	■
	Hollister-Stier		Formalin (0.8% Formaldehyd)		●
	Dr. Sasse	5	Formaldehyd	1	
	Trolab	004	Formaldehyde	2	
Furacin → Nitrofural					
Hexachlorocyclohexane → Lindane					
Hexachlorophene (WHO) (Ph)	Hermal	19	Hexachlorophen	0.5	□
	Hollister-Stier		Hexachlorophene	0.5	▶

	Manufacturer	Code	Name	Value
Hexamethylenetetramine	Trolab	0101	Hexachlorophene	1
Hexylresorcinol	Trolab	1007	Hexamethylenetetramine	1
Histadyl → methapyrilene hydrochloride	Dr. Sasse	Am29	Hexylresorcin	0.5
Hydrazine sulfate	Trolab	0802	Hydrazine sulfate	1
Hydroquinone	Dr. Sasse	L34	Hydrochinon	1
	Trolab	0800	Hydroquinone	1
Hydroquinone monobenzylether	Trolab	1001	Hydroquinone monobenzylether	1
p-Hydroxybenzoate → Paraben				
Isobutyl-p-aminobenzoate	Trolab	1102	Isobutyl-p-aminobenzoate	5
Isopropylmyristate	Trolab	1201	Isopropyl myristate	20
Lanolin alcohols	Hermal	2	Adepslanae	100
	Hollister-Stier		Woolwax alcohol	30
	Dr. Sasse	4	Wollwachsalkohol-derivate	30
Lindane	Trolab	0020	Wool alcohols	30
Mafenide (WHO)	Trolab	0702	Lindane, hexachlorocyclohexane, gamexane	1
	Hermal	4	Aminomethylbenzolsulfonamid	10
Malathion	Dr. Sasse	3	Mafenid	10
Menthol	Trolab	0701	Malathion	0.5
2-Mercaptobenzimidazole	Hermal	16	Menthol	1
2-Mercaptobenzothiazole (MBT)	Trolab	1006	2-Mercaptobenzimidazole	1
	Hermal	14	Mercaptobenzothiazole	2
	Hollister-Stier		Mercaptobenzothiazole	1
Mercury	Dr. Sasse	14	Mercaptobenzothiazole	2
	Trolab	1010	Mercaptobenzothiazole (MBT)	1
	Hollister-Stier		Mercuric chloride, ammoniated	5
	Dr. Sasse	7	Hydrargyr. bichlorate	0.1
	Trolab	0602	Ammoniated mercury	1
	Trolab	0603	Mercury	0.5

Table 17a—continued

Test substance	Firm	No.	Trade name	Test concentration (%)	Vehicle, etc.
Merthiolate → Thiomersal					
Methapyrilene hydrochloride	Hollister-Stier	L33	Histadyl	1	▶
p-Methylaminophenol	Dr. Sasse	0801	p-Methylaminophenolsulfat	1	■
	Trolab		p-Methylaminophenolsulfate(metol)	1	◀
2.2'-Methylene-bis(-4-methyl-6-tert.-butylphenol)	Dr. Sasse	G24	2.2-Methylen-bis(-4-methyl-6-tertiar-butyl-phenol)	1	■
Methylparaben	Hollister-Stier		Paraben, Methyl	3	▶
Methylsalicylate	Hermal	18	Methylsalicylat	2	□
Metol → p-methylaminophenol					
Morpholinylmercaptobenzothiazole	Trolab	1015	Morpholinylmercaptobenzothiazole (MOR)	1	◀
Neomycin (sulfate) (WHO)	Hermal	7	Neomycinsulfat	5	□
	Hollister-Stier		Neomycin sulfate	20	▶
	Dr. Sasse	1	Neomycinsulfat	20	■
	Trolab	0010	Neomycin sulfate	20	◀
Nickel sulfate	Hermal	28	Nickelsulfat	2	□
	Hollister-Stier		Nickel sulfate	2.5	▶
	Dr. Sasse	12	Nickelsulfat	2	■
	Trolab	0003	Nickel sulfate	2.5	◀
Nitrofural (WHO)	Hollister-Stier	M39	Furacin	0.2	▶
	Dr. Sasse		Nitrofurazon	1	■
Nitrofurazon → Nitrofural					
o-Nitro-p-phenylene diamine	Trolab	0301	o-Nitro-p-phenylenediamine	2	◀
Nupercaine → Cinchocaine					
Oil of laurel	Hermal	15	Lorbeerol	2	□

Substance	Supplier	No.	Name	Conc.
Pantocaine → Tetracaine				
Pellidol (DAB)	Dr. Sasse	13	Pellidol	2
Penicillin-G-sodium	Dr. Sasse	M40	Penicillin-G-Natrium	(1 mill I.E.)
Peru balsam	Hermal	8	Perubalsam	10
	Hollister-Stier		Balsam of Peru	25
	Dr. Sasse	20	Perubalsam	25
	Trolab	0008	Balsam of Peru	25
Petrolatum → Vaseline				
Phenol-formaldehyde resin	Trolab	0901	Phenol formaldehyde resin	5
Phenyl-β-naphtylamine	Trolab	1003	Phenyl-β-naphthylamine	1
N-Phenyl-cyclohexyl-p-phenylenediamine	Hermal	13	N-Phenyl-cyclohexyl-p-phenylen-diamin	2
	Dr. Sasse	G27	N-Phenyl-cyclohexyl-p-phenylendiamin	1
	Trolab	1012	Phenylcyclohexyl-p-phenylenediamine	1
p-Phenylenediamine	Hermal	24	p-Phenylenamin	1
	Hollister-Stier		Paraphenylendiamine	1
	Dr. Sasse	6	p-Phenylendiamin	1
	Trolab	0005	p-Phenylendiamine (PPD)	2
Phenylisopropyl-p-phenylendiamine	Trolab	1004	Isopropylaminodiphenylamine (IPPD)	0.1
Phenylmercury salt	Dr. Sasse	19	Phenylmercuriborat	0.025
	Trolab	0601	Phenylmercuric nitrate	0.05
Potassium dichromate	Hermal	26	Kaliumdichromate	0.1
	Hermal	21	Kaliumdichromate	0.5
	Hollister-Stier		Potassium dichromat	0.5
	Dr. Sasse	2	Kaliumdichromat	0.5
	Trolab	0001	Potassiumdichromate	0.5
Primin (synthetic)	Trolab	0000	Primula	1 μg Primin
Procaine (WHO)	Hermal	6	Procain	2
	Dr. Sasse	M36	Procainhydrochlorid	1
	Trolab	0400	Procaine chloride	3
Propylparaben	Hollister-Stier		Paraben, propyl	

Table 17a—continued

Test substance	Firm	No.	Trade name	Test concentration (%)	Vehicle, etc.
Pyribenzamine → Tripelennamine					
Resorcinol	Hermal	17	Resorcin	0·5	□
	Dr. Sasse	AM31	Resorcin	2	■
	Trolab	0302	Resorcinol	2	◄
Sterosan → Chlorquinaldol					
Surfacaine → cyclomethycaine					
Turpentine	Hermal	23	Terpentin	10	□
	Hollister-Stier		Turpentine	10	▶
	Dr. Sasse	18	Terpentinol	10	■
	Trolab	0009	Turpentine peroxides	0·3	⊙
Tetraethylthiuram disulfide (TETD)	Trolab	1016	Tetraethylthiuramdisulfide (TETD)	1	◄
TCSA tetrachlorsalicylanilide (Ph)	Trolab	0102	Tetrachlorsalicylanilide	0·1	◄
Tetracaine (WHO)	Dr. Sasse	M38	Pantocainhydrochlorid	1	■
	Trolab	0402	Amethocaine chloride	1	◄
Tetramethylthiuram disulfide (TMTD)	Hermal	12	Tetramethylthiuramdisulfid	2	□
	Hollister-Stier	17	Tetramethylthiuramdisulfid	2	▶
	Dr. Sasse		Tetramethylthiuramdisulfid	2	■
	Trolab	1011	Tetramethylthiuramdisulfide (TMTD)	1	◄
Tetramethylthiurammonosulfide	Dr. Sasse	G22	Tetramethylthiurammonosulfid	1	■
	Trolab	1008	Tetramethylthiurammonsulfide (TMTM)	1	◄
Thiomersal	Hollister-Stier	0600	Merthiolate sodium	0·1	▶
	Trolab		Thimersal	0·1	◄
Toluenediamine	Hermal	25	p-Toluylendiamin	1	□
	Trolab	030	p-toluenediamine sulfate	1	◄
Tribromsalan (Ph)	Hollister-Stier		Tribrominated salicylanilide	1	▶
	Trolab	0103	Tribromosalicylanilide	1	◄

Tribromosalicylanilide → Tribromsalan					
Triethylenetetramine	Trolab	0905	Triethylenetetramine (epoxy curing agent)	0.5	◄
Tripelennamine (WHO)	Hollister-Stier		Pyribenzamine	2	►
Tricresol phosphate (TCP)	Trolab	0904	Tricresyl phosphate (tritolyl phosphate)	5	◄
Vaseline	Hermal	1	Vaseline	100	□
	Hollister-Stier		Control (Petrolatum)	100	►
Vioform iodochlorhydroxyquinoline					
Wool alcohols → Lanolin alcohols					
Zinc ethylene-bis(-dithiocarbamate)	Trolab	0700	Zineb(ethylenebis (dithiocarbamate) zinc	1	◄
Zinc diethyldithiocarbamate	Trolab	1009	Bis(diethyldithiocarbamate)zinc (ZDC)	1	◄
Zinc dibutyldithiocarbamate	Trolab	1019	Bis(dibutyldithiocarbamato)zinc (ZBC)	1	◄

a Mixtures of test substances see Table 4.

Table 17b. Other test substances (chemicals)

Abietic acid, 5% pet.
Alantolactone (Helenin), 0.1% pet.
Alcohol, ethyl, etc. 10% aq.
Allylglycidylether, 0.25% MEK
p-Aminoazotoluene, 1% pet. or MEK
p-Aminobenzoic acid and esters, 5% pet.
p-Aminodiethylaniline, 1% pet.
p-Aminophenol, 2% pet.
p-Aminosalicylic acid (PAS), 2% pet.
Ammonium persulfate, 1% aq.
Anethole, 2% alc, or pet.
Aniline, 1% pet.
Aniline dyes, 5% pet.
Anthraquinone, 2% pet.
Arylsulfonamide formaldehyde resin (nail polish), 10% MEK
Aureomycin, 5% pet.
Azo dyes, 1% pet. or MEK
Bacitracin, 20% pet.
Balsam of Canada, 25% pet.
Balsam of pine, 20% MEK
Balsam of spruce, 20% MEK
Balsam of Tolu, 10% alc.
Beeswax, 30% pet. and olive oil ana.
Benzalkonium chloride, 0.1% aq.
Benzaldehyde, 5% pet. or 10% alc.
Bensetone chloride, 0.1% aq.
Benzidine, 2% MEK
Benzyl alcohol, 5% pet. or alc.
Benzyl cinnamate, 5% pet. or 10% alc.
Bergamot oil, 2% pet.
Beryllium chloride, 2% aq.
Bitter almonds, oil of, 10% O.O.
p-t-Butylcatechol, 1% and 2% pet.
n-Butylglycidylether, 0.25% MEK
p-t-Butylphenol, 2% pet.
Carbamide-formaldehyde, 10% pet.
Carbowax, as is
Cassia, oil of, 2% pet.
Cedarwood oil, 10% pet.
Cetylalcohol, 30% pet. and olive oil ana.
Cetylpyrimidine, 0.1% aq.
Chloramine, 0.5% aq.
Chloroacetamide, 0.1% aq.

Chloramphenicol, 5% pet.
Chlorhexidine, 0.5% aq.
Chloroacetophenone, 0.1% alc.
p-Chloro-*m*-cresol, 1% pet.
Chloroquine sulfate, 5% aq.
p-Chloro-*m*-xylenol, 1% pet.
Cincaine, 5% pet.
Cinnamic acid, 10% pet.
Cinnamic alcohol, 10% pet.
Cinnamon aldehyde, 1% alc.
Citral, 2% pet.
Citronella, oil of, 2% pet.
Cloves, oil of, 2% pet.
Coniferylbenzoate, 2% pet.
Coumarin, 10% 0.0.
n-Cresylglycidylether, 0.25% MEK
Dammar resin, 20% alc. or pet.
2,4-Diaminophenol (amidol), 2% pet.
Dibutylphthalate, 5% pet.
N,N',-dibutyl-*p*-phenylenediamine, 1% pet.
Dichloronitrobenzene, 0.1% acetone
Diethylaminosalicylate, 2% pet.
Diethylenetriamine, 1% MEK or pet.
Diethyl-*p*-phenylenediamine, 1% pet.
Diethylstilbestrol, 1% alc.
Dihydrostreptomycin, 0.1% pet.
Dihydroxydichlorodiphenylsulfide, 1% alc.
Dihydroxydiphenyl, 0.1 pet.
Dimethylaniline, 1% pet. or alc.
Dinitrophenylaniline, 1% pet.
Dioctylphthalate, 5% pet.
Dioctyl-*p*-phenylenediamine, DOPD, 2% pet.
Dioxane, 1% aq.
Dipentene, see Limonene
Diphenyl-*p*-toluidine, 2% pet.
Di-*o*-tolylbiguanidine, 2% pet.
Dodecylgallate, 1% pet.
Dyes, organic, 2% pet.
Eosin, 50% pet.
Epoxy diluents (reactive), 0.25% MEK
Erythromycin, 1% pet.
Essential oils, 1% pet.
Eucalyptus, oil of 2% pet.
Eugenol, 5% pet.
Explosives, 1% pet.
Fluorescein, 10% pet.
Framycetin, 20% pet.
Fuchsin, 1% pet. or alc.
Geraniol, 5% pet.
Glucocorticosteroids, 25% pet.

Glutaraldehyde, 1% aq.
Gold sodium thiosulfate, 0.1% aq.
Halogenated salicylanilides, 1% MEK
Hexamethylenetetramine, 2% pet. or aq.
Hexylresorcinol, 2% pet.
Iodine, 0.5% alc.
Isoeugenol, 5% pet.
Kanamycin, 20% pet.
Lavender, oil of, 2% pet.
Lemon, oil of, 2% pet.
Lemon grass, oil of, 2% pet.
Lidocaine (Xylocaine), 5% pet.
d-Limonene (dipentene), 2% pet.
Maneb, 2% pet.
Melamine-formaldehyde, 10% alc.
2-Mercapto-6-nitrobenzothiazole, 2% pet.
Methyl orange, 2% pet.
Methylmethacrylate, 2% pet.
Methyl salicylate, 2% pet.
Metol(methyl-*p*-aminophenol sulfate), 2% aq.
Mirbane oil, 10% O.O.
α-(and β-)Naphthol, 0.1% pet. or 1% alc.
Naphthylamine, 2% alc.
α,β-Naphthylthiourea, 2% pet.
Neroli, oil of, 2% pet.
Octylgallate, 1% alc.
Optical whiteners, 0.1–1% pet.
Orange, oil of, 2% pet.
Pentachlorophenol, 1% alc.
Pentadecylcatechol, 0.1–1% MEK
Peppermint, oil of, 2% pet.
Phaltan, 0.1% pet.
Phthalic acid or anhydride, 1% alc.
Phenothiazines, 1% aq. or pet.
Phenylethanol, 5% pet.
Phenylglycidylether, 0.25% MEK
Phenyl salicylate (Salol), 1% pet.
Phosphosesquisulfide, as is
Picric acid, 1% aq.
α-Pinene, 15% olive oil
Piperazine derivatives, 5% aq.
Pitch, 5% pet.
Platinum chloride, 1% aq.
Potassium persulfate, 5% aq.
Pyrethrum, 2% pet. or 5% MEK
Pyrocatechol, 2% or aq.
Pyrogallol, 1% pet. or aq.
Quaternary ammonium salts, 0.1% aq.
Quinine, 1% aq.
Rubber chemicals, 2% pet.

Saccharin, as is
Salicylaldehyde, 2% pet.
Sodium diethyldithiocarbamate, 2% pet.
Sorbic acid, 5% pet. or aq.
Spearmint, oil of, 2% pet.
Storax, oil of, 2% pet.
Storax, 2% pet.
Streptomycin, 0·1–1% aq.
Sulfonamides, 5% pet.
Terramycin, 3% pet.
Tetracyclines, 5% pet.
Thiamine, 10% aq.
Tobacco, as is
p-Toluidine, 2% pet.
Trichlorocarbanilide, TCC, 2% pet.
Tricresyl phosfate, 10% MEK
Triethanolamine, 2% aq.
Trinitroanisol, 1% pet.
Trinitrophenol, 1% aq.
Trinitrotoluene, 1% pet.
Urea-formaldehyde, 10% pet.
Usnic acid, 1% pet.
Vanilla, as is
Vanillin, 10% pet.
Venice turpentine = larch turpentine, 20% pet.
Vitamin B_1, 10% pet.
Vitamin B_6, 10% pet.
Xanthocillin, 10% pet.
Xylocaine, 2% aq.
Zineb, 2% pet.
Ziram, 2% pet.
Zirconium, sodium zirconium lactate, 0·1% aq. intraderm.

Table 17c   Other test substances (products)

Adhesive tape, as is
Antibiotics (topical) 10% pet.
Antihistamines (topical), as is
Antimycotic agents (topical), as is and 25% pet.
Ballpoint-pen dye, as is
Barrier cream, as is and 50% pet.
Carbon paper, as is, wetted with acetone
Cold wave, 2% aq.
Cutting oil, 10% and 50% aq.
Deodorant, stick, as is
Drilling oil, as is and 50% 0.0.
Dye, food, as is 2% pet.
Fruit (orange, citrus peel), as is (possibly primary irritant)

Furniture polish, 10% and 50% acetone or olive oil
Glue, 1% –20%, aq., acetone, ethanol, pet.
Hair lacquer, as is
Hair lotion, as is and 50% O.O. or ethanol
Hand lotion, as is and 50% pet.
Ink, as is
Insect spray, as is (after evaporation)
Latex, as is after evaporation of irritant solvent
Lipstick, as is
Lubricating oils, as is and 50% O.O.
Mascara, as is
Nail polish, as is or arylsulfonamide-formaldehyde resin
Paints, as is and 10% and 50% O.O.
Perfume, as is (i.e. 10% in alc.)
Photographic chemicals, 1% and 10% aq.
Photographic paper, as is
Plant, leaf, flower, pollen, bulb, as is
Plastic, as is
Shampoo, 5% aq.
Spice, as is and oils of, 5% ethanol
Sunscreen, as is
Thinner, as is and 50% acetone
Toilet water (eau-de-Cologne), as is (i.e., perfume 1% alc.)
Toothpaste, as is and 50% pet.
Varnish, 10% and 50% O.O. or acetone
Wood, exotic, dry sawdust
Wood, pine and spruce; balsams of pine and spruce (sawdust false-negative)

10. Flow Chart for Patch Testing

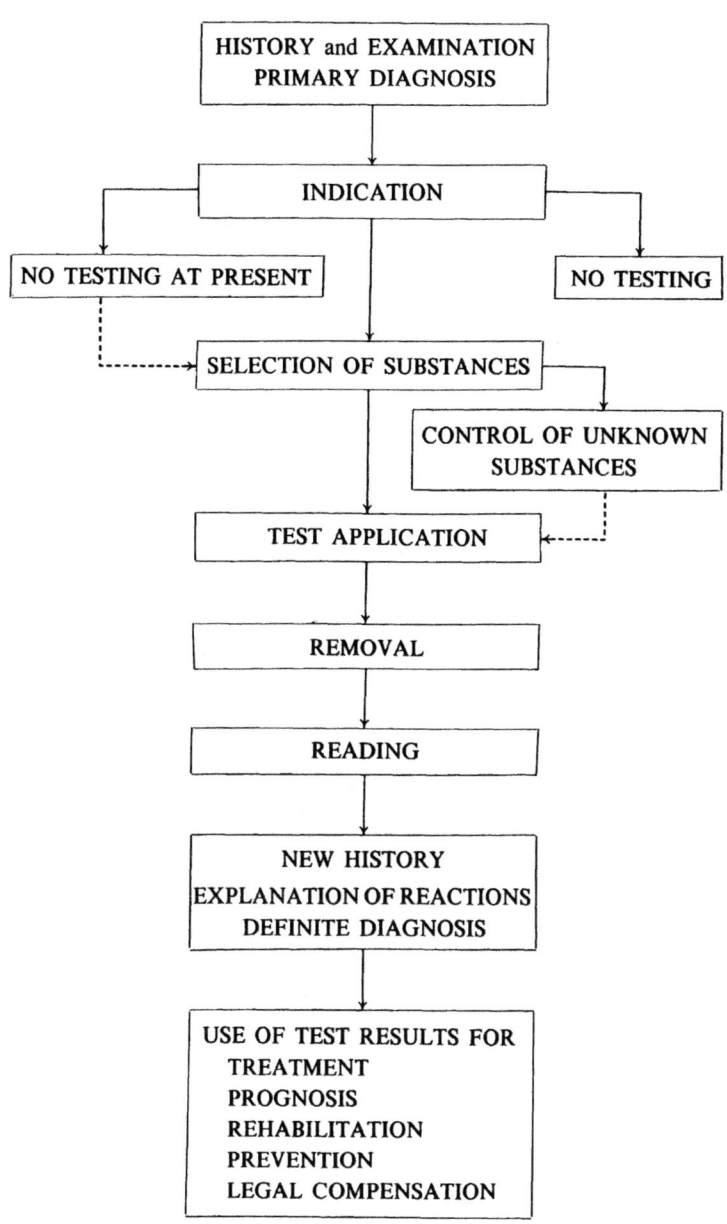

11. Bibliography

ADAMS, R. M.: *Occupational Contact Dermatitis.* Philadelphia and Toronto: J. B. Lippincott Company. 1969.

BANDMANN, H.-J., DOHN, W.: *Die Epicutantestung.* Munich: J. F. Bergmann. 1967.

BLOCH, B.: Ekzem und Überempfindlichkeit. *Schweiz. med. Wschr.* 4, 629 (1923).

COOKE, R. A.: Quoted by COCA, A. F.: Studies in specific hypersensitiveness. *J. Immunol.* 7, 193 (1922).

FISHER, A. A.: *Contact Dermatitis.* Philadelphia: Lea and Febiger. 1973.

FOUSSEREAU, J., BENEZRA, C.: *Les eczémas allergiques professionnels.* Paris: Masson et Cie. 1970.

FREGERT, S.: *Manual of Contact Dermatitis.* Copenhagen: Munkgaard. 1974.

FREGERT, A., HJORTH, N., MAGNUSSON, B., BANDMANN, H.-J., CALNAN, C. D., CRONIN. E., MALTEN, K., MENEGHINI, C. L., PIRILÄ, V., WILKINSON, D. S.: Epidemiology of contact dermatitis. *Trans. St. John's Hosp. derm. Soc.* 55, 17 (1969).

HJORTH, N.: Eczematous allergy to balsams. *Acta derm.-venereol. (Stockh.) Suppl.* 46, 1961.

HJORTH, N., FREGERT, S.: Contact dermatitis. In: *Textbook of Dermatology,* edited by ROOK, A., WILKINSON, D. S., EBLING, F. J. G., Sec. edition, Oxford and Edinburgh: Blackwell Scientific Publications. 1972.

IPPEN, H.: *Index Pharmakorum.* Stuttgart: Georg Thieme. 1968.

JADASSOHN, J.: *Verhandl. Deutsch. Dermat. Gesellsch. Fünfter Congress (1895),* 1896, 103.

MALTEN, K. E., ZIELHUIS, R. L.: *Industrial Toxicology and Dermatology in the Production and Processing of Plastics.* Amsterdam, London, New York: Elsevier Publishing Company. 1964.

RÖMPP, H.: *Chemielexikon.* Stuttgart: Franckh'sche Verlagshandlung. 1962.

SCHULTHEISS, E.: *Gummi und Ekzem.* Aulendorf i. W.: Editio Cantor. 1958.

SCHULZ, K. H.: Berufsdermatosen. In: *Dermatologie und Venerologie* Bd. V/1. Herausgeg. v. GOTTRON, H. A., SCHÖNFELD, W., Stuttgart: Georg Thieme. 1963.

SULZBERGER, M. B.: *Dermatologic Allergy.* Springfield: C. C. Thomas Publ. 1940.

WILKINSON, D. S., FREGERT, S., MAGNUSSON, B., BANDMANN, H.-J., CALNAN, C. D., CRONIN, E., HJORTH, N., MAIBACH, H. J., MALTEN, K. E., MENEGHINI, C. L., PIRILÄ, V.: Terminology of contact dermatitis. *Acta derm.-venereol. (Stockh.)* 50, 287 (1970).

12. Index

12.1 General

12.2 Chemicals

Pages in *italics* refer to substances when used at testing

75

77

G. Plewig, A. M. Kligman
Acne
Morphogenesis and Treatment

R. G. Freeman, J. M. Knox
Treatment of Skin Cancer
(Recent Results in Cancer Research, Vol.11)

L. Goldman
Laser Cancer Research
(Recent Results in Cancer Research, Vol.4)

N. Hunziker
Experimental Studies on Guinea Pig's Eczema
Their Significance in Human Eczema

In preparation (1976):

O. Braun-Falco, S. Lukacs, H. Goldschmidt
Dermatological Radiotherapy

GPSR Compliance

*The European Union's (EU) General Product Safety Regulation (GPSR)
is a set of rules that requires consumer products to be safe and our
obligations to ensure this.*

*If you have any concerns about our products, you can contact us on
ProductSafety@springernature.com*

In case Publisher is established outside the EU, the EU authorized
representative is:

Springer Nature Customer Service Center GmbH
Europaplatz 3
69115 Heidelberg, Germany

Batch number: 09635029

Printed by Printforce, the Netherlands